SITTING ON THE JOB

A PRACTICAL SURVIVAL GUIDE FOR PEOPLE WHO EARN THEIR LIVINGS WHILE SITTING

SCOTT W. DONKIN, D.C.

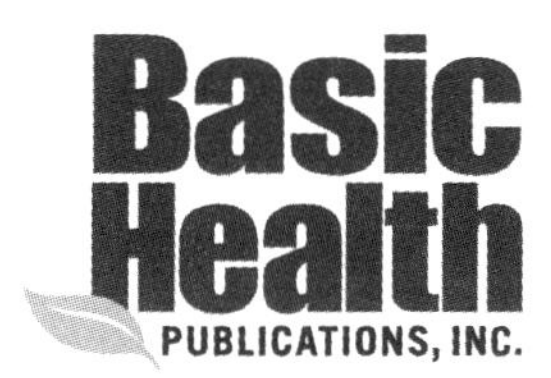

The information contained in this book is based upon the research and personal and professional experiences of the author. It is not intended as a substitute for consulting with your physician or other healthcare provider. Any attempt to diagnose and treat an illness should be done under the direction of a healthcare professional.

The publisher does not advocate the use of any particular healthcare protocol but believes the information in this book should be available to the public. The publisher and author are not responsible for any adverse effects or consequences resulting from the use of the suggestions, preparations, or procedures discussed in this book. Should the reader have any questions concerning the appropriateness of any procedures or preparation mentioned, the author and the publisher strongly suggest consulting a professional healthcare advisor.

Basic Health Publications, Inc.
8200 Boulevard East
North Bergen, NJ 07047
1-201-868-8336

Library of Congress Cataloging-in-Publication Data
Donkin, Scott W.
Sitting on the job : a practical survival guide for people who earn their livings while sitting / Scott W. Donkin.
p. cm.
Previously published: Lincoln, Neb. : Parallel Integration, 1987.
Includes bibliographical references and index.
ISBN 1-59120-013-X
1. Offices—Health aspects. 2. Sitting position—Health aspects.
3. Human engineering. 4. Stress management. 5. Human mechanics. I. Title.
RC965.O3 D65 2002
613'.088'651—dc21
2002010316

Typesetter/Book design: Gary A. Rosenberg
Cover design: Mike Stromberg

Printed in the United States of America

10 9 8 7 6 5 4 3 2 1

Contents

To my wife, Mary Pat,
whose constant support and incredible patience
helped transform these thoughts and ideas into reality.

She taught me, by example,
that life and work should be fun
and that everyone should be given
the opportunity to realize this concept.

- Δ Governments, companies, and businesses rise or fall, advance or recede, in direct relation to the quality, enthusiasm, and dedication of their most valuable asset . . . their human resources.
- Δ Providers of goods and services need to sincerely foster comfort, health and well-being, enthusiasm, and creativity within their priceless human resources in order to prosper during this rapidly changing and competitive time in history.
- Δ The human resources must take responsibility for their own health and fully utilize their skills and talents to help meet and exceed the goals and visions of their employers.
- Δ Team effort is essential to survive and prosper.

Foreword

Office work was once seen as a nice, safe occupation for a woman to pass time in before she got married. Now the truth is out. Far from being an incidental way to earn some extra pin money, most office jobs are filled with women who have to support themselves and their families. It is the largest sector of the workforce, and the one that employs the most working women: one out of every three working women is a clerical worker.

And office work is not necessarily safe. With the increased use of office computers, or video display terminals (VDTs), more and more clerical workers are getting injured on the job. The number of worker's compensation and disability cases filed, and won, is on the rise. Back injuries, painful wrist inflammations requiring surgery, and eye problems are typical. The injuries cost employers in payments and time lost, and cost employees in suffering and sometimes in permanent injuries.

Clerical work is also stressful. Workers with the most stressful jobs are not air-traffic controllers or high-level executives, as most people think. According to the federal government, it's VDT workers.

Many VDT operators are closely monitored. Their every keystroke is counted. They have to make a quota or risk losing their jobs. Even trips to the bathroom are counted. As one woman told me, "I feel as if I'm in constant battle with my job, and it always wins. I used to like going to work, but now it's a nightmare."

The good news is that it doesn't have to be this way. Offices need not be booby-trapped. Chairs and tables and machines can be made adjustable and comfortable, to fit our bodies, instead of torture them. Workloads can be better organized, and breaks can give office workers a chance to catch their breath and rest their eyes.

The first step is learning how things ought to be, and that's where *Sitting on the Job* comes in. This book tells you what kind of workstation is best, and how to use it. And it provides suggestions for breaks and exercises to mitigate the inevitable stress and strain you experience even if you have the best workstation design in the world. If you follow Dr. Donkin's advice, you'll find yourself feeling better. And you'll find you can do your job better too.

The next step is getting your employer to make it possible for you to follow the advice in *Sitting on the Job.* A long history of fighting for occupational health and safety in this country tells us that we have to push for change. We've seen this time after time, with chemical toxins, asbestos, and machine-induced injuries, informed employees, working with organizations like 9to5, both educate employers and can hold them accountable to a standard that says we are entitled to safe, healthy, and comfortable workplaces.

We all stand to gain. Employers will have more productive employees who perform better on the job and spend less time out on sick leave. And employees will feel better and be much less likely to get hurt working, even just sitting, on the job.

Karen Nussbaum, Executive Director
9to5, National Association of Working Women

Preface

The concept for *Sitting on the Job* was conceived in 1982. It was published after six years of writing and rewriting. Fifteen printings later, it has now been revised for you. When *Sitting on the Job* was first published, most people had never heard of ergonomic principles. This was before highly adjustable office chairs, keyboards, monitors, and headsets became widely available, and before taking your wallet out of your back pocket when sitting became popular. However, there is still a tremendous need to understand how to set up your workstation properly and how to service the physical and mental demands of modern work. These concepts can also be applied to other aspects of your life. With longer workdays and more dependence on computers, *Sitting on the Job* is more important than ever before.

Millions of people who earn their livings while sitting needlessly endure excessive pain, stress, and strain during their work and in their lives. Many people feel that these are necessary evils in today's "civilized," "sophisticated," and "technological" society. I believe that, although these complaints are common, they are not normal. The physical and emotional effects of pain, strain, and negative stress represent signals or cries for help. First, we must admit that these problems exist. Then we can discover and implement positive solutions.

One particular case comes to mind. One of my patients suffered a severe neck and back injury as a result of an automobile accident. I had been treating her for quite some time for the effects of this injury. She had experienced relief from many of her original complaints, but she still suffered severe headaches at times. Our treatment would alleviate the headaches but they would continue to recur. A pattern began to emerge. She would have fewer symptoms during weekends and holidays. We finally discovered that, during the course of her work duties, she had to frequently look through the lower lens of her bifocal eyeglasses in order to inspect information that appeared on a video display terminal. The viewing screen was positioned too high for her and she had to repeatedly tilt her head backward to see the screen, thus aggravating her injured neck and contributing to her recurring headaches. Once the appropriate workstation changes were implemented, she recovered and was released from care for the effects of this injury. We also discovered that her productivity and job satisfaction dramatically improved. Similar situations among my patients were common.

A system needed to be created to discover how an individual feels about his or her workplace in order to determine if conditions exist in the workstation, in the work environment, or in the individual that interfere with the worker's ability to efficiently, consistently, and accurately perform his or her tasks, and to do so without pain, discomfort, and stress. An organization known as Peak Performance Health and Safety (PeakHealthandSafety.com) was created to provide this service to companies and businesses. The concepts, procedures, and services provided by Peak Performance Health and Safety are described in Appendix D.

One of the primary solutions is to help people understand the nature of their work and work environment so they can learn how to achieve greater comfort and productivity at their workstations and how to counteract the possible negative effects involved with the type of work they perform.

This book was written with this goal in mind. It is fully illustrated to enable you to easily capture and understand important concepts. The figures were developed without gender so as not to imply sexual bias.

It would be impossible to describe and explain every situation in everyone's unique work setting. The content, design, and format of this book is intended to give you concepts with which you can understand what changes need to be made in your work setting and in your work habits, and why these changes are essential for you and your work.

A well-designed chair cannot achieve its maximum effect unless you, the user, understand how to make it fit your body and use it in the manner for which it was designed. The same is true for well-designed workstations, equipment, and other instruments you use in the performance of your tasks. They can't help you unless you understand their proper function and use them appropriately.

This book describes practical methods designed to help you create a better fit between your work environment, your workstation, and your unique body. This book also gives you practical techniques to reduce stress, counteract the effects of long periods of sitting, and thus enhance the quality of your life.

Acknowledgments

This book, throughout its creation, has been a team effort even though some participants didn't know they were members of the team.

Joseph J. Sweere, D.C., DABCO, has been my friend and mentor throughout the writing, editing, and publishing of this book. He enthusiastically contributed his valuable time and vast knowledge to improve the quality and accuracy of the entire book. He always gave much more than I expected. He did this in spite of an incredibly busy schedule, the extraordinary demands he places upon himself, and the enormous requests from his profession to help create, research, and develop programs and procedures to help industry preserve and enhance the quality of their most valuable asset . . . their human resources.

Jan Kelley Weinberg contributed her tremendous creative talent and organizational skills to edit and illustrate this book in a manner that is attractive, easy to read, and understand. Jan made concepts from the written material clearly visible through the illustrations. She did not hesitate to make many sacrifices and was always enthusiastic throughout the creation of this book.

John and Elizabeth Laugen provided priceless input for the organization of this book and the development of an efficient, systematic approach to help organizations, which employ people who perform their tasks while sitting, to identify conditions in the work environment and workstations that interfere with the health, productivity, and job satisfaction of their workers; to systematically implement solutions to preserve and enhance the quality of their most valuable asset . . . people; and to systematically evaluate the effect of these solutions.

Thomas M. Wolff, APR, is the editor of *Staying Well,* a bimonthly newsletter published by the Foundation for Chiropractic Education and Research. He researched and organized the information published in *Staying Well.* Many of his concepts and researched material were used in this book. I am grateful to have this newsletter available and to be able to present some of the information in this book. I highly recommend his newsletter to everyone interested in their health and well-being.

Rani Karen Lueder, principal of Humanics, a human factors consulting firm in Encino, California, contributed her incredible knowledge of ergonomics to help me accurately present the sections on how people can create a better fit between their unique bodies and their workstations and why this is essential. During my research, she recommended appropriate books and sent valuable articles so that facts would be well documented.

Mark Hirschfeld, a consultant with Selection Research, Inc., in Lincoln, Nebraska, contributed his valuable time to read the original manuscript. He helped me understand that human resources are every organization's most valuable asset. Caring and being sincerely interested in the individuals that comprise the workforce creates an environment of enthusiasm and cooperation that encourages people to fully contribute their individual talents to effectively and productively surpass the minimum requirements for producing goods and services. Companies, businesses, and governments need this type of environment to survive and prosper during these rapidly changing times. Mark completely redesigned the tools used by Peak Performance Health and Safety so that meaningful data could be extracted from the studies performed for companies, businesses, and government agencies.

Tom Cebuhar and Sue Bernt at Lincoln Tour and Travel enthusiastically provided a section of their office to perform the pilot study by Peak Health & Safety (see appendix D for info). Sue read the original manuscript of this book and gave me valuable feedback about its contents.

Jan Beckwith, creator and president of Body Flex, Inc., read the original manuscript and enthusiastically provided safe and effective exercises that are explained in this book. She has been a constant supporter of this material.

Jolene Anderson deciphered more than 200 pages of my handwritten scribble and typed it neatly and accurately into manuscript form. I believe she is the only one who could have done it. She neatly organized the original and modified forms used in the Lincoln Tour and Travel pilot study. Whenever I requested her services, she sacrificed evenings and weekends to meet my needs.

The doctors and staff of the Chiropractic Associates and my partner, David Lauer, and his wife, Kelly, were understanding and supportive while I was revising this book. They allowed me to fulfill this goal and helped me continue to provide quality care to my patients.

Sandra Wendel, from Editorial Services, Inc., in Omaha, Nebraska, edited the original manuscript and helped me understand the valuable contribution that this book could make.

Larry Pelter, an energy conservationist at Lincoln Electric System, and member of their safety committee, contributed his time to read the original manuscript and provided valuable input. Larry, Kerry Jones, and Tom Chapman invited me to give lectures and slide presentations to almost all of the office workers and engineers at Lincoln Electric System. Their feedback helped me organize an effective lecture and slide presentation to help people understand the concepts in this book so they could apply them in their work and in their lives.

Charlene Henninger, Madelein Matis, Ph.D., Larry McPhillips, Marvin Schlegel, John Sullivan, Lorrie Vojtech, and Sandy and Dean Weinmeister also read the original manuscript. All of the people who read the original manuscript represented a group of individuals with varied talents and occupations. All had one thing in common: they earned their livings while sitting. They contributed their time to read the original manuscript and gave me invaluable feedback as to how it helped them make improvements in their workstations and habits to enhance the quality of their health, well-being, and their work. They helped make the information in this book easier to read and understand.

One look at the references in the back of this book will tell you that there are many more contributors. These doctors, scientists, and researchers used their talents to fulfill their desire to help their fellow humans discover meaningful information. Many of their facts, concepts, and ideas have been integrated into this book. They certainly deserve a great deal of credit for the guidance this book provides to help its readers become happier, healthier, and more productive in their chosen occupations, and enhance the quality of their lives.

Introduction

This Is an Exciting Day for You!

Yes, this is indeed an exciting day for you because you have discovered information that will help you not only to survive, but also to thrive in your chosen occupation. This book will outline and explain information about you and your body as well as fundamentals of your workstation and its environment. You will discover some of the effects your work has on your body and learn how you can reduce or eliminate problems that can affect your health, well-being, job performance, and job satisfaction.

You will learn how stress affects you and practical techniques to turn its negative effects into positive action. You will also learn how essential it is to properly fit your body into your workstation as well as change your workstation to fit your body.

This book will provide you with a great deal of knowledge about you and your work and will offer solutions of which you can take advantage. You will be encouraged to take action to work for your benefit and to be consistent with these recommendations in order to achieve maximum results. Knowledge, action, enthusiasm, and consistency are the keys you need to unlock and open the doors to a healthier, happier, and more productive future in your chosen occupation.

Your workstation and environment may seem like a man-made jungle that can feel as imposing and stressful as living in a natural jungle. One can survive and thrive in a natural jungle, if its rules or laws are understood and obeyed. If these rules are ignored, one is sure to perish. Less life-threatening, but every bit as important to you, is knowing and understanding the laws that govern the physical and mental demands of your work. Your ability to survive and thrive in your chosen occupation is directly dependent on your knowledge and understanding of these laws and your ability to make them work to your advantage.

Many employers are aware of much of the information we are about to share with you and will be pleased to learn that you are participating in a positive growth experience. Knowledgeable employers understand that whatever you do to help yourself be more comfortable and healthier will also help you become more enthusiastic, more productive, and a greater asset to the company or business.

First, you must know and understand your body and how it functions. With this knowledge, you will realize the value of the changes you can make to effectively combat the forces that may be causing you problems during your work activities. You really have nothing to lose and much to gain, so let's begin our journey to find the knowledge that will allow you to change things you probably didn't know you could.

1

Your Body

Your body is a miracle of engineering, physics, chemistry, and electronics. All of these combine to form what humankind has not been able to duplicate and probably never will.

The core of your physical body is the nervous system. The brain, spinal cord, and peripheral nerves regulate all of the functions of your body. Virtually every cell in your body has a nerve supply that communicates information to and from your brain. In fact, it has been said that if you took everything away from the body except the nerves, the remaining nerve network would create an exact replica of the human being. You would even be able to recognize the individual! When your parents were children, it was believed that when the heart stopped the individual was no longer living. Modern science now recognizes that physical life ends when the brain dies. The brain is the source of all the energy that travels through the nervous system; human life is not possible without this nerve energy (see Figure 1.1).

Nerves are very delicate and sensitive, so protection is provided in the form of calcium-laden bones. The skull protects the brain, and the spinal vertebrae protect the spinal cord (see Figure 1.2). A layer of protein liquid (cerebrospinal fluid) surrounds the brain and spinal cord to provide nutrition and to act as an effective shock absorber. There is little movement between the bones of the skull, but the neck and back must be flexible to allow smooth and graceful motion; therefore, a series of bones called vertebrae are provided to allow this motion and still give protection. The vertebrae are stacked on top of one another like building blocks and are separated by donut-shaped cushions called discs. The discs hold portions of the vertebrae together and provide shock absorption for the body in standing and sitting postures.

Spinal nerves leave the spinal cord through openings between the vertebrae in order to serve all the parts of the body (see Figure 1.3). The spinal bones must be anchored together but still allow motion, so the body has strong, but elastic ligaments (see Figure 1.4). These ligaments help tie the bones together while the muscles, by their ability to contract and relax, actually move the bones. This is

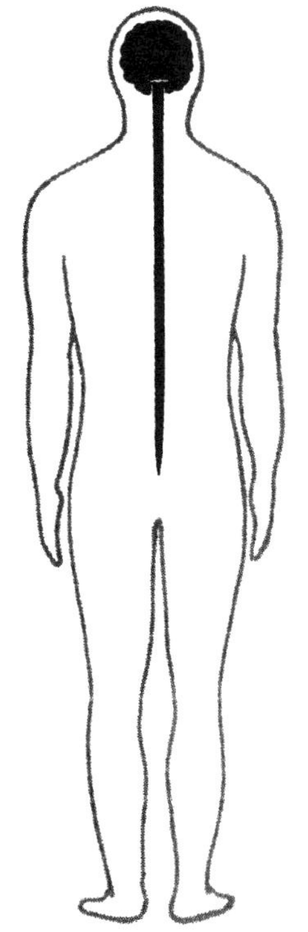

FIGURE 1.1. The brain and spinal cord control and regulate the human body.

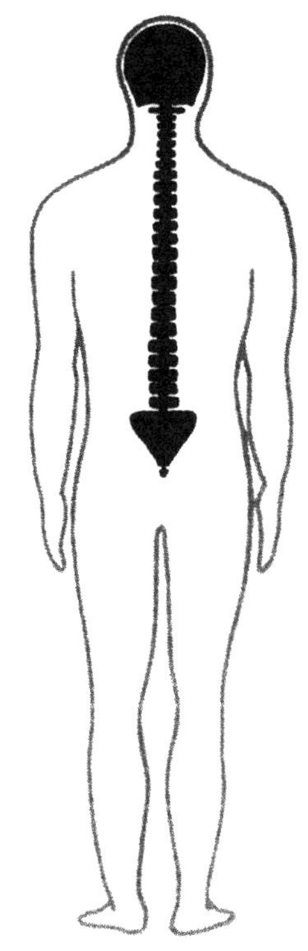

FIGURE 1.2. The brain is protected by the skull, and the spinal cord is protected by vertebrae that form the spine.

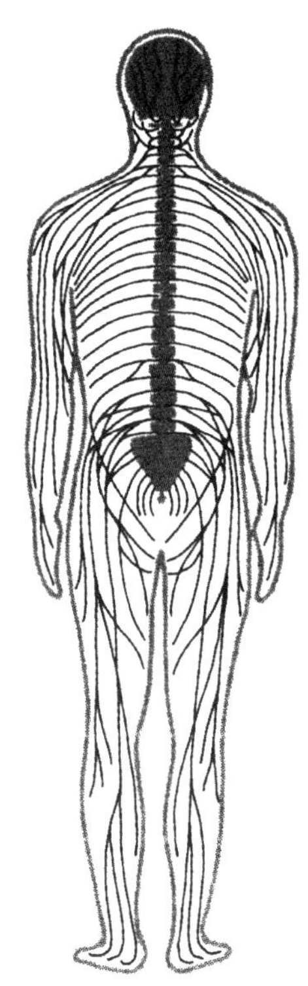

FIGURE 1.3. Spinal nerves leave the spinal cord through openings between the vertebrae to serve all parts of the body.

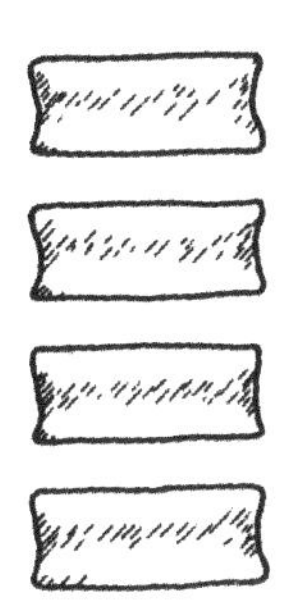
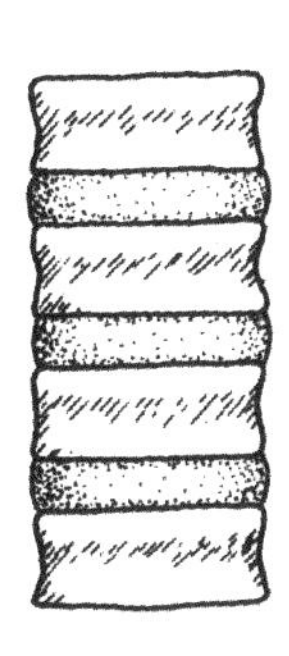
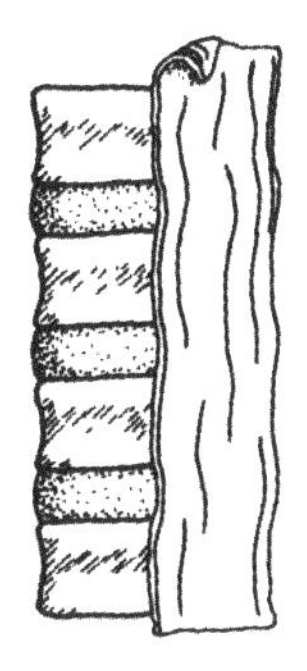
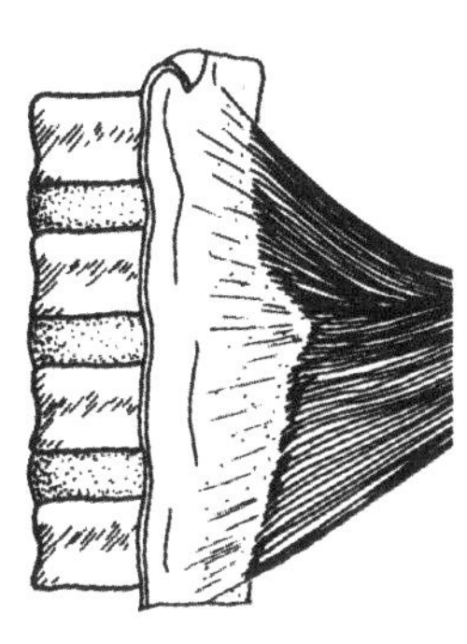

FIGURE 1.4. The spine is made up of vertebrae and discs that are bound together by ligaments and muscles.

true not only for the vertebrae, but also for the bones and joints of the arms, hands, legs, and feet. Many muscles narrow into tendons, which anchor into the bones for extra leverage. The bones provide the levers, the ligaments hold the bones together, and the muscles move the bones. All of this action is controlled by the nervous system.

Basic Body Mechanics

Your body must be able to move from one place to another. Your legs with their joints and powerful muscles make this possible (see Figure 1.5). Your feet and legs provide the foundation for your body. The legs attach through the hip sockets to the pelvis, which, with the sacral bone, provides the foundation or base for the spine and the rest of the body.

The physical body could be viewed as a vehicle or machine and must obey the universal laws of physics and engineering. This is where balance becomes important. The laws of gravity reign over all physical structures and this includes the human body. Your upper body must be balanced over your legs; otherwise, you would tend to fall over. Ideally, your spine would be straight up and down (vertical or plumb) with your shoulders equally balanced over your body (see Figure 1.6). Such isn't always the case, and it is this quality of uniqueness about your body that you must become aware of.

Most of us deviate to some extent from perfectly normal balance, but the extent to which you vary from normal can be the extent to which you experience physical stress and strain that can eventually become aches and pains. For example, if you have a fallen arch on one foot, or if you have one leg shorter than the other, your hips and pelvis will become distorted and your total body balance will be affected (see Figure 1.7). When the nervous system is working

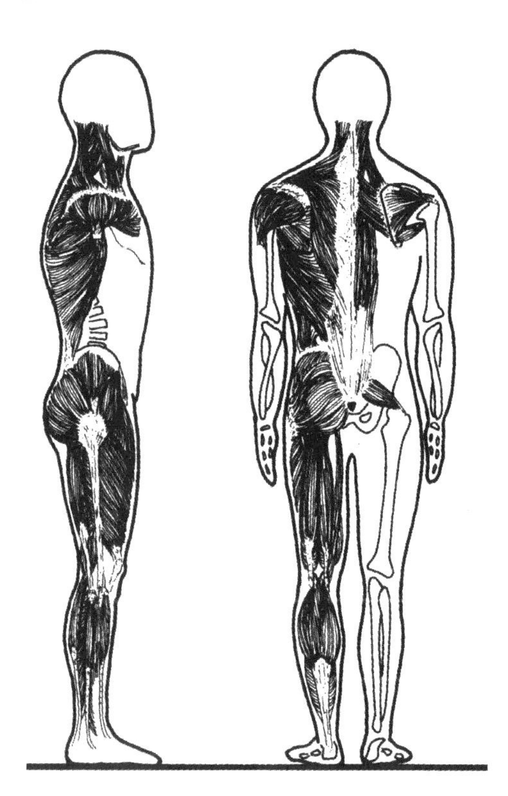

FIGURE 1.5. Muscles, through contraction and relaxation, allow us to move and help us to maintain balance and posture.

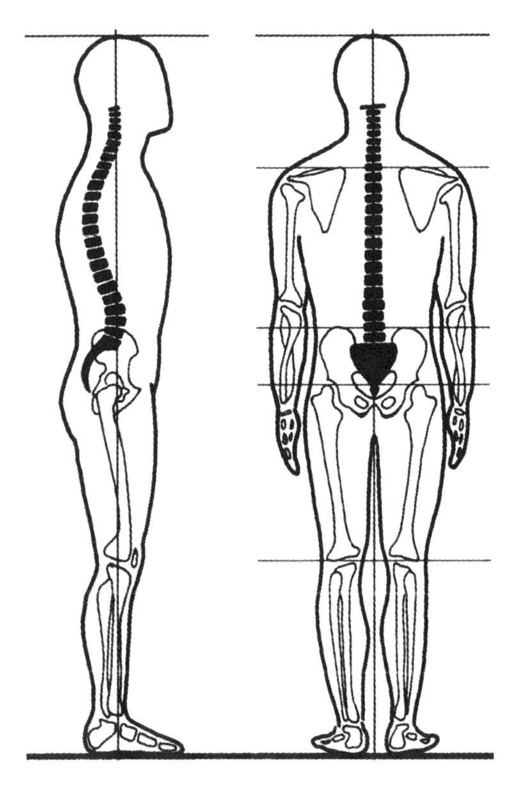

FIGURE 1.6. Ideally, the spine should be vertical when viewed from behind and S-shaped when viewed from the side.

properly, the body has a marvelous ability to adapt for imbalance by twisting and turning other body parts to compensate. If, however, vertebrae become misaligned or lodged in a position that is other than their normal alignment during this process of compensation, or as a result of trauma or stress, nerve irritation can result. The term commonly used to describe this phenomenon is subluxation. Subluxation is abnormal position and/or motion of bones at a joint that is less than dislocation, but significant enough to crowd, stretch, or otherwise irritate the nerve fibers, which, in this case, exit between the vertebrae (see Figure 1.8). Subluxations become a source of spinal weakness and instability, muscle spasm, and nerve irritation, which produce such symptoms as pain, burning, numbness, and tingling.

Here is where another law of nature comes in to play. A structure that bears

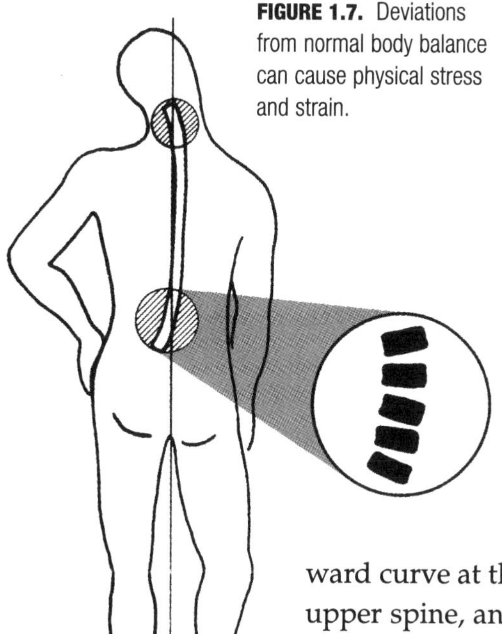

FIGURE 1.7. Deviations from normal body balance can cause physical stress and strain.

more stress and strain tends to wear out faster. This is similar to the uneven wear you see on your car tires if the wheels are unbalanced or out of alignment. These same forces or laws of nature affect you and your body. The objective here is to make you aware that these laws exist and show you how they can affect you and your body.

When looking at the body from a side view, the spine should normally have four curves. There should be a backward curve at the tailbone, a forward curve at the lower spine, a backward curve at the upper spine, and a forward curve at the neck. The two forward curves should counterbalance the two backward curves to allow the entire trunk to remain balanced over the center of gravity (see Figure 1.9). This S-shaped configuration is designed to provide a means of shock absorption much like a coiled spring absorbs shock. These forward and backward curves are normal and desirable in both the standing and sitting postures. If the spinal curves are reduced, producing a "ramrod" alignment, or are bowed too much, producing a "swayback" or "hunchback," biomechanical stress and strain is created. You should, therefore, work to preserve these normal curves in both the standing and sitting postures.

It would be easier to sit in conventional chairs if our bodies were square, boxlike, and all the same size, but that just isn't the case. We are designed with

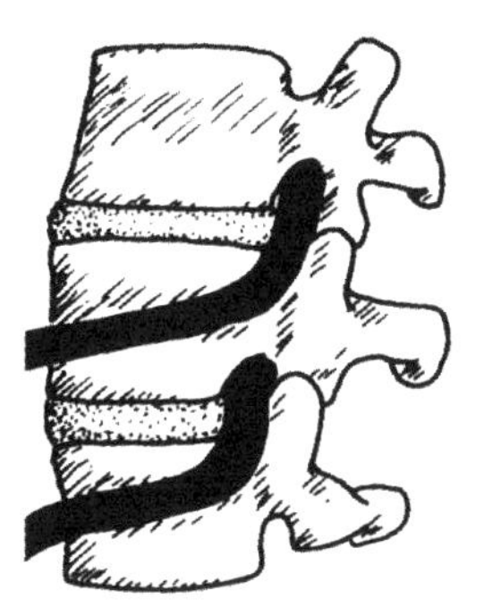

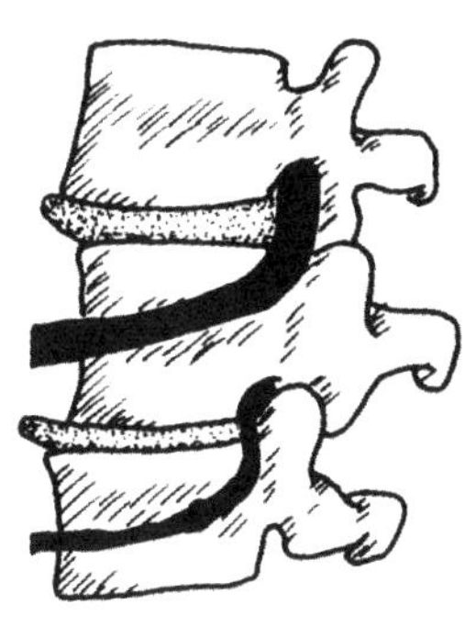

FIGURE 1.8. Vertebrae that are not properly aligned or that do not move normally can cause strain, nerve irritation, and abnormal wear in the joints over time.

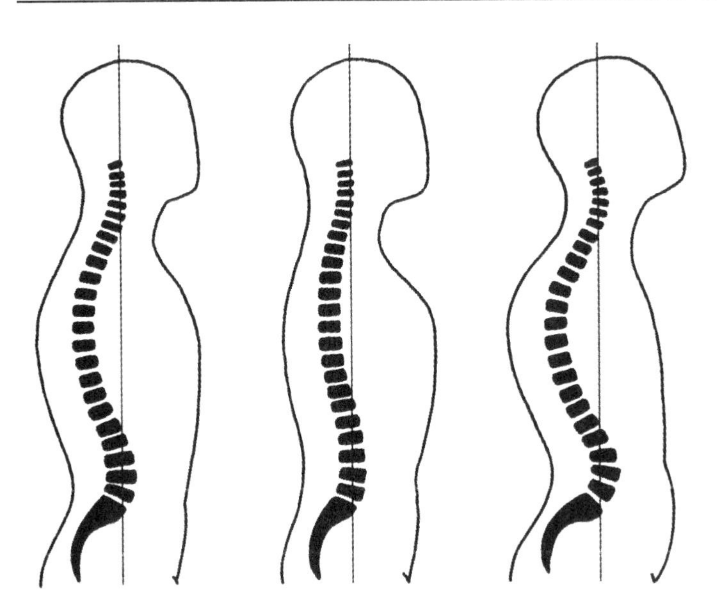

FIGURE 1.9. Normal spinal curves (left). Reduced spinal curves (center). Increased spinal curves (right).

curves, bends, and in different sizes and shapes. These contours do not fit well into a straight chair. As the saying goes, "You cannot fit a round peg into a square hole." Ideally, a chair should fit and support the unique shape and contour of the body (see Figure 1.10). The extent to which a chair does not provide this fit and support is the extent to which the body experiences physical strain. It would be to your benefit to adjust or modify your chair to fit your body as much as possible. If you have a straight-backed chair, you may need to fit a specially designed supportive pillow in the space between the chair and the natural forward curve of your lower back (see Figure 1.11). If you have a well-designed contoured chair, you need to make sure it fits your spinal curves properly. If the backrest is too low or too high, it can add to back strain and put pressure on the wrong parts of your body. You will learn more about proper sitting positions from the explanations in Chapter 2 that illustrate how to fit your body into your workstation and how to alter your workstation to fit your unique body.

Habits and Time

At this point you may be asking, "Why should I take action to improve my posture and consistently adjust my chair to fit my body?" Another law of human nature is that we are creatures of habit and, as time passes, we actually become

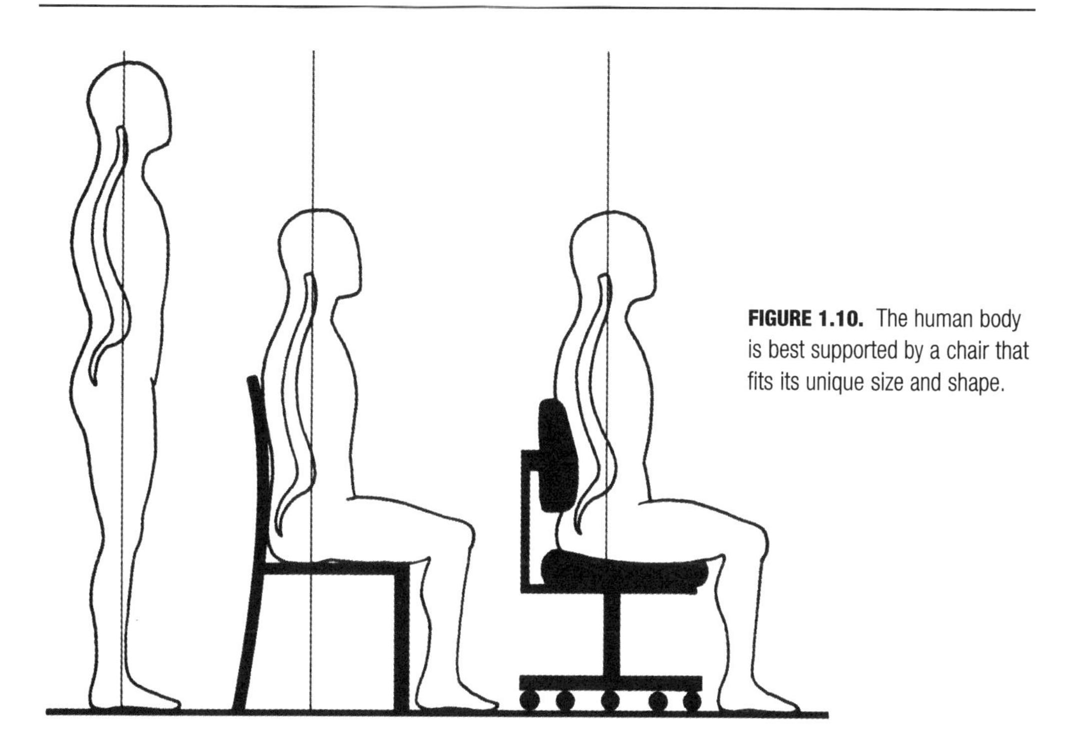

FIGURE 1.10. The human body is best supported by a chair that fits its unique size and shape.

"creatures of our habits." In other words, our bodies tend to conform to the positions and postures our bodies assume most often. Our bodies also try to accommodate and conform to the activities we perform and the manner in which we perform them.

The ligaments and other connective tissues that hold our bones together have what is referred to in engineering terms as both "elastic" and "plastic" properties. The elastic property of these tissues can spring back to their original form when a stretch or movement is completed. The plastic property of these tissues has a puttylike character and tends to remain at a tension or position that the tissues are in most often. If you spend the majority of your workday slumped at your desk with your head flexed forward or are always turning in one direction, the connective tissues will allow your body to eventually conform to those abnormal positions. Unknowingly, you are "training" your body to become unbalanced.

There is another important point you must know about the joints and connective tissues before you can understand the solution to this problem. Let's zoom in on one of your joints. A joint is formed where two adjacent bones meet

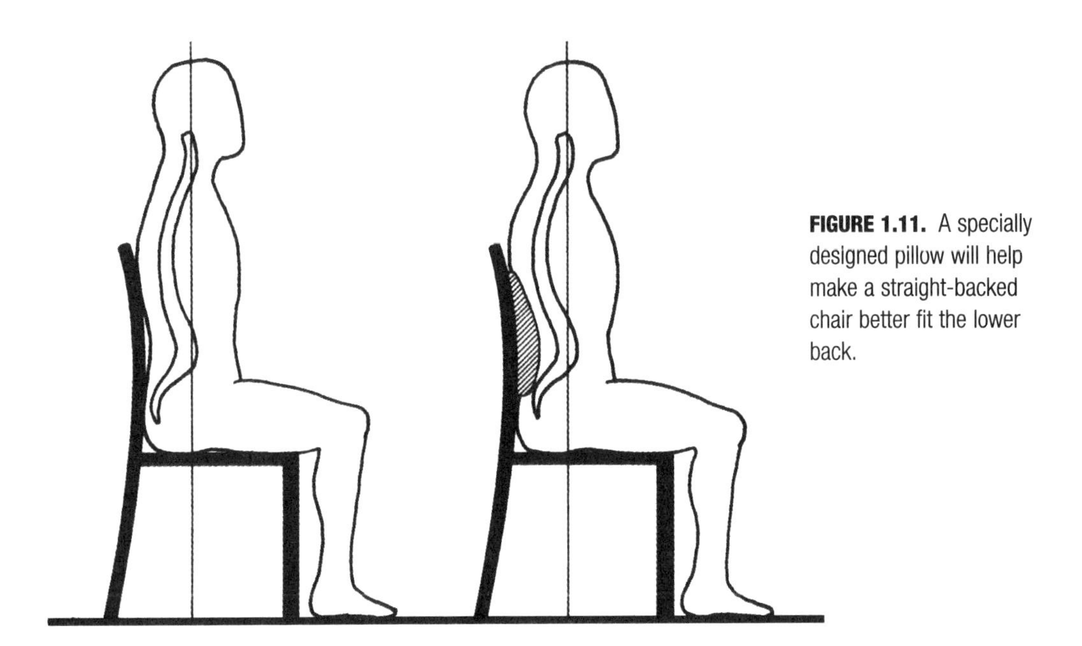

FIGURE 1.11. A specially designed pillow will help make a straight-backed chair better fit the lower back.

and are held together by ligaments. These bones have a certain range in which they can move (see Figure 1.12). Forced movement outside of this range produces "sprain" and/or "dislocation." The catch is that the joint must move through its total range of normal movement or it will tend to be "limited to only the range that it is used to moving." This law of nature says, "If you do not use it, you will lose it!"

If you have ever had a cast on your leg for a broken bone, you will understand this principle. When the cast is first removed from your leg, you can hardly move the joints. They are stiff and the muscles are weak from lack of use. If you work hard to rehabilitate the leg by frequently stretching the joint and exercising the muscles, you may regain full function of movement and strength.

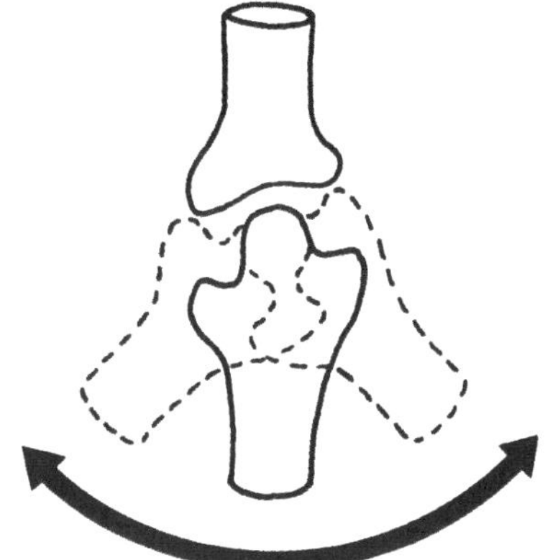

FIGURE 1.12. Two bones that come together to form a joint have a certain range in which they can move.

Now you know that your body tends to conform to the positions and postures it assumes most often, and the body will restrict joint motion to the range that it is used. It takes time for these changes to affect you because these processes of conformity and restriction progress slowly. You may not become aware of a problem until it becomes serious in terms of pain, muscle spasm, tension, or fatigue, due to imbalance, misalignment, restriction, and nerve irritation.

A middle-aged man consulted me one day for a neck and shoulder problem. He explained that his neck and shoulder started to bother him several years earlier, but he didn't think much of it. He was an avid golfer, but swinging the clubs became painful. Instead of having his problem examined and treated, he gradually quit playing golf. He said he lost interest in the game because it made him uncomfortable. As time passed, other activities involving reaching with his arms and shoulders and turning his neck bothered him, so he limited his activities even further. He finally decided to seek help when he could no longer look over his shoulder to back his car out of the driveway and couldn't raise his arm high enough to apply underarm deodorant.

It took time, treatment, and hard work to correct the underlying problem, which we discovered was a neck and shoulder injury from a fall he had suffered. He was ultimately able to regain more than 80 percent of the function of his neck, shoulder, and arm. Along with the physical improvement was an improvement in his attitude and work productivity. This typical case illustrates how limited movement creates increasing restriction, which over time greatly interferes with body function and the ability to perform routine daily activities such as work, sleep, and recreation.

Time can be a friend or an enemy. If you are not doing anything about maintaining good posture or exercising your body to keep its mobility and vitality, time is your enemy, and you are likely to suffer the consequences in one form or another. If you strive to obtain and maintain good postural habits and keep your body and its joints flexible and properly conditioned, time can be your friend.

Advantages of Sitting Properly

You may be asking yourself, "If slumping in my chair is so bad for me, why does it feel better at times?" Slumping is the body's instinctive attempt to take strain and tension away from muscles that are working to maintain prolonged postures (see Figure 1.13). The problem may be a result of sitting in an ill-fitting chair, sitting too long in one posture without movement, sitting in an unbal-

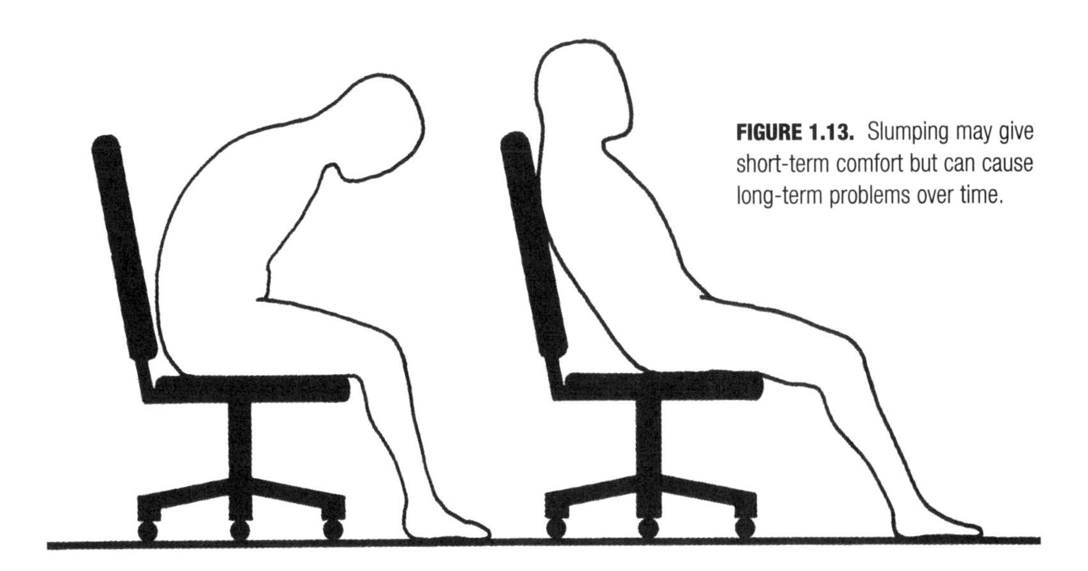

FIGURE 1.13. Slumping may give short-term comfort but can cause long-term problems over time.

anced posture, or some type of spinal misalignment or condition that is causing the muscles to work harder or to become fatigued. Poor muscle condition or tension from cumulative negative stress can also be important factors. The body tries to relieve strained muscles by slumping, placing a greater burden on the spine. Shifting the burden from the muscles to the spine creates greater pressure on the discs between the vertebrae. The normal S-shaped curve of the spine is designed to effectively bear the weight of the body while the muscles are designed to hold and maintain the spine in this position. When these curves are altered while sitting, pressure on the discs is greatly increased. Spinal imbalance or vertebral misalignment can add to disc pressures and create back problems significant enough to require professional care. Remember that physical structures bearing greater stress and strain wear out faster. In this case, your spine is more susceptible to degeneration.

Thus, long-term slumping postures can give you significant problems that overshadow the short-term muscular relief they provide. In fact, long-term slumping ultimately requires greater muscular effort and creates increased tension and restriction of movement. In addition, slumping postures tend to encourage shallow breathing, which can cause fatigue. You need to move about in your chair and assume various postures during the workday and leaning forward toward your work surface is probably one of them. Acquiring the habit of slumping forward a majority of the time is not in your best interest. I believe that it is by far better to use the contour and positioning of your chair to support your spine in its erect posture and use relaxation and exercise techniques to keep your muscles healthy. You will learn more about these techniques later in this book.

Now that you have a basic understanding about body mechanics and how your body functions, you may still be wondering what this has to do with your job. You were employed to perform certain physical and mental tasks so that your employer could provide a product or service to consumers. In the private sector, companies must produce this product or service efficiently, competitively, and for a profit. Otherwise, they could not exist. In the government sector, the operation should run efficiently and effectively with taxpayers' dollars and within a restrictive budget. You were chosen because your employer had confidence that you could perform certain tasks that were essential to the operation of the business or company. You should take pride in being selected for your ability to effectively perform those tasks to which you were assigned.

You must, however, be able to perform these tasks efficiently, accurately, and consistently in order to preserve your employment and receive the monetary rewards and other benefits that result from your talents and services. If you and your coworkers could not perform the designated tasks efficiently, accurately, and consistently, the company or business could not thrive and you would risk losing your job.

Your ability to perform your tasks with greater comfort and ease will not only increase your productivity, but also increase your job satisfaction and make a healthier and more pleasant environment for you to work. Less stress and strain at work preserves your energy for leisure time enjoyment and for your home, personal, and family life as well.

So read on to the next chapter about your workspace and learn how you can preserve your body and still perform your tasks at maximum efficiency and comfort. It is important to you!

2

Your Workspace

Look around your workstation. What do you have? You probably have a chair, desk, light, possibly a computer terminal with a keyboard, a typewriter, telephone, calculator, pens, pencils, other tools, paper, and probably books, magazines, and catalogs. You may have family pictures or personal belongings that you are fond of that make your workstation a little more like home. So here you are, the operator of this workstation. At this workstation, you must efficiently perform tasks that are vital to the operation of the company or business. Just like the pilot of an airplane, you have your tools and instruments in front of you. However, is your "instrument panel" arranged properly for your body and your task?

You may have been hired to replace someone who had worked at this workstation before you. Suppose that person was left-handed and you are right-handed, or they were six feet, one inch tall and you are five feet, four inches tall. Suppose this person was lazy, inefficient, and left the workstation in a mess. You, on the other hand, want to be comfortable and productive so things will be better for you and your employer. At this point, the workstation certainly isn't going to suit you and your body. You may make some changes instinctively, but unless you know how things are supposed to fit, you may miss the mark a bit and still experience some problems.

The best way to make the workstation and you fit together is to look at it as though this were your first day on the job (see Figure 2.1). It's kind of like a fresh start. After all, you are gaining a different perspective about your work and it may make your job seem new again. We will start at the foundation, your chair, and work upward.

Your Chair

If you use the same chair every day, properly adjusting it to fit your body may require little daily effort. If you use a different chair each day or someone else uses your chair during another shift (see Figure 2.2), you need to adjust it each time you use it, as you would adjust your car seat, steering wheel, and mirrors if someone else had used your car. If you don't, over a period of time, you and your body will pay the price.

The objective is to make your chair fit the length, size, and contours of your body for maximum support and comfort. Your body, like your fingerprints, is unique and deserves a personally modified chair that will allow you to sit comfortably for many hours each day. Study the recommended sitting postures in Figure 2.3. What is considered the "perfect sitting posture" is somewhat undetermined for all humans and varies according to the type of work you do, so the

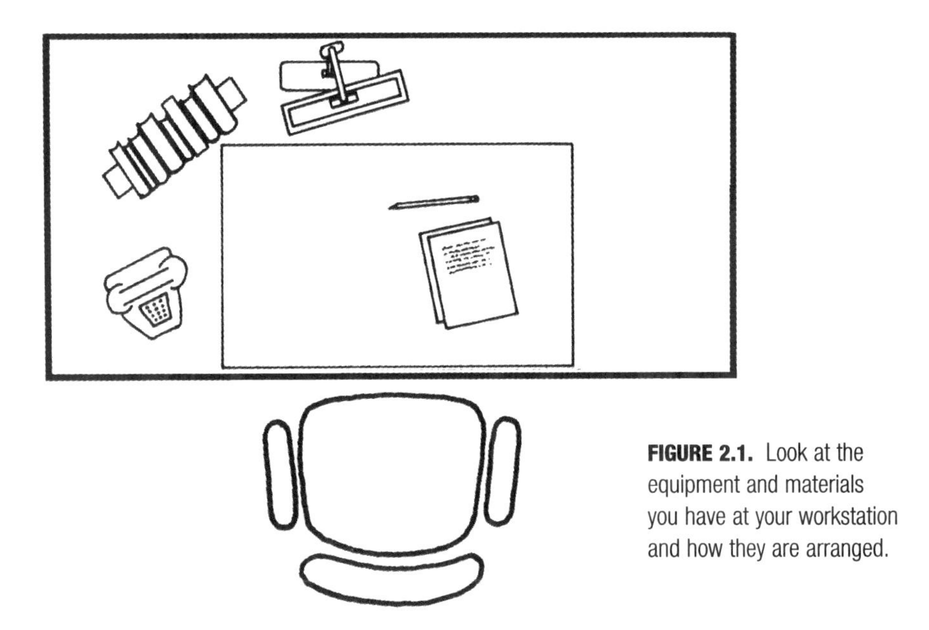

FIGURE 2.1. Look at the equipment and materials you have at your workstation and how they are arranged.

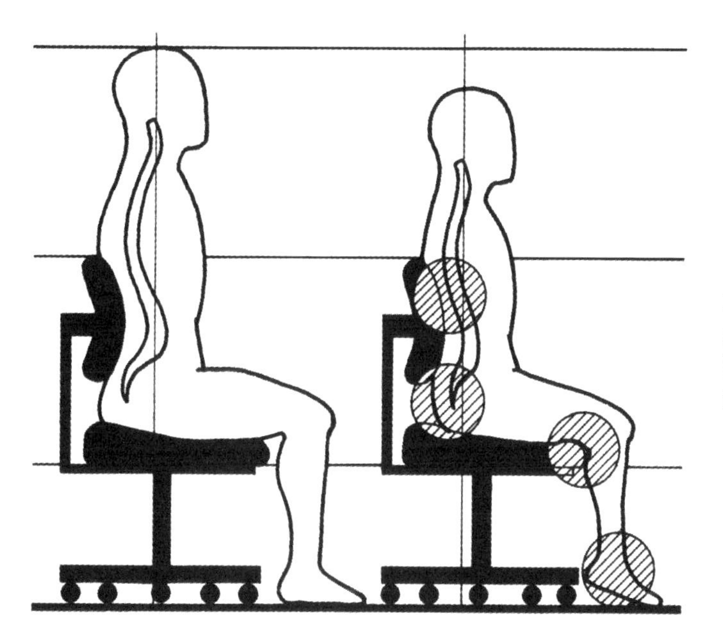

FIGURE 2.2. The chair on the right needs to be adjusted to fit this worker's body. Is your chair adjusted to fit your body?

basic guidelines are illustrated in the figures. You should use the posture or postures that make you feel most comfortable, but still provide support while you perform your tasks. Do not confuse support and comfort with thick, soft, overstuffed chair cushions. If you sink into your chair more than an inch, your

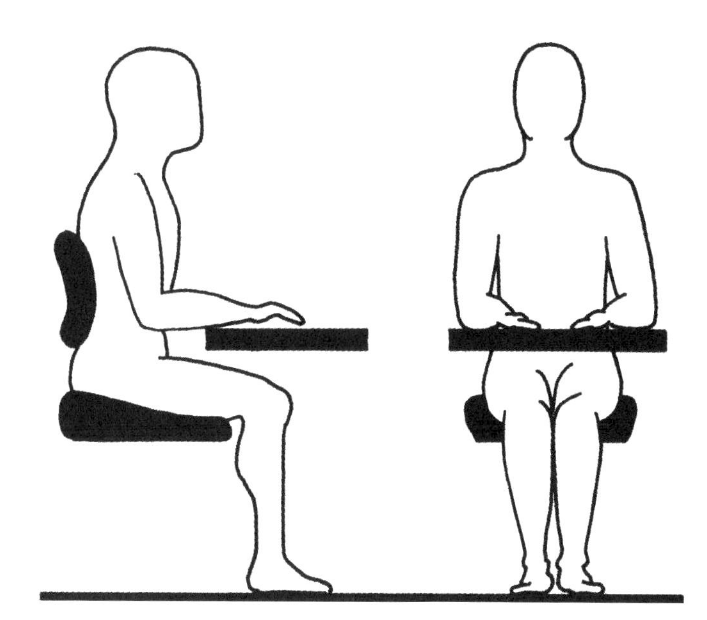

FIGURE 2.3. Well-supported and balanced sitting postures.

body tends to collapse into the cushions and cannot obtain the proper support that it needs. Your chair should be lightly padded so the cushion can evenly distribute the weight of your body. Fabric upholstery on the cushions helps prevent slipping and sliding, and reduces the amount of effort required to maintain your appropriate sitting postures.

Before 1900, it was thought that the perfectly correct posture for work performed in the sitting position was in a chair that rigidly supported the spine at a right angle to the legs with the knees also bent at right angles. Actually, this position quickly becomes uncomfortable, and it is almost impossible to perform your tasks in this one position. Pressure soon develops in the back, buttocks, and thighs when holding this position, making it difficult to concentrate on your job. When your thighs are at right angles to your back, the curve of your lower back tends to straighten, unless you have and use a properly contoured backrest support. The usual compensation for lack of proper backrest support is to take the weight of the upper body off of the lower back by slumping forward. This slumping posture increases pressure on the discs between the vertebrae and ultimately makes the muscles and ligaments of your back work harder, thus increasing their tendency toward strain. If you constantly lean to the right or to the left at your workstation, you may also be adding further stress and strain to your body. You are now beginning to understand how the postures and positions in which you hold your body can be making you uncomfortable.

You can remove a great deal of pressure and strain from your body by adjusting the backrest position and tension height, chair height, and the angle of the "seat pan" so that your tailbone and pelvis tip forward. If you have an adjustable chair, use it to your advantage.

The type of work you perform determines how you should adjust your chair (see Figure 2.4). If the task requires reading and writing at a desk, you need to lean forward, so the seat pan should be tilted forward, up to 15 degrees, so the thighs can angle downward and help preserve the natural curves of your spine and reduce the pressure on your thighs. The seat pan can be adjusted slightly higher when it is tilted forward. Some recent studies have indicated that a slightly higher seat pan height may reduce disc pressures in the spine. If you primarily operate a computer terminal with a keyboard, you do not need to lean forward as much, so the seat pan can be tilted slightly backward, about 5 or more degrees from level depending on the design of the chair, to enable

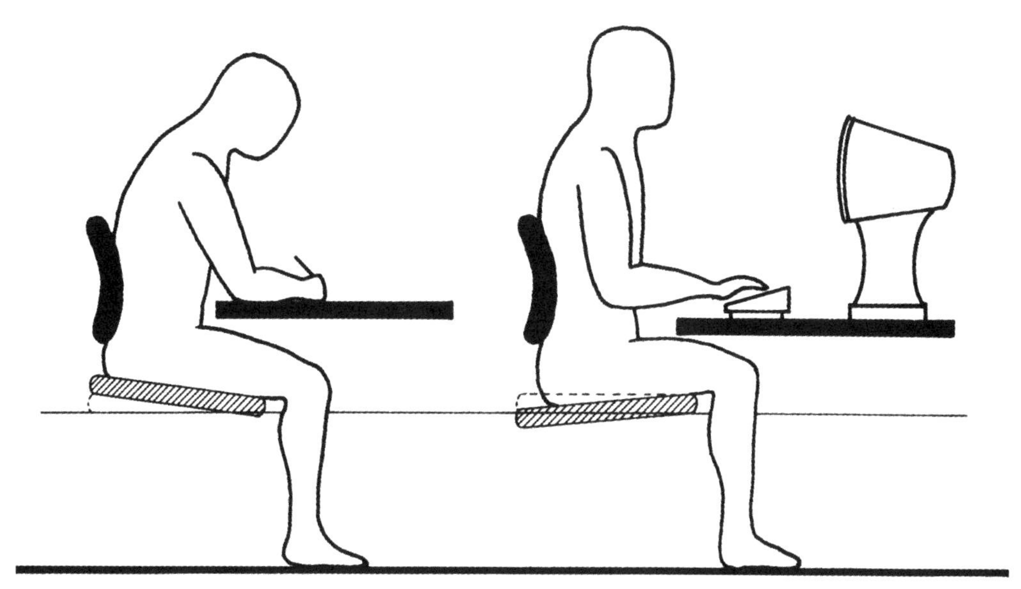

FIGURE 2.4. Adjusting the chair's seat pan may greatly improve comfort.

you to take advantage of the lumbar support in the backrest. Studies performed by Drs. Grandjean, Hunting, and Piderman in Zurich, Switzerland, revealed that most video display terminal operators preferred and used postures in which they leaned backward in a position similar to that of a car driver.

At this point, a word of caution is in order. Do not tilt the seat pan forward to the degree that you feel you are sliding out of the chair. Do not tilt the seat pan backward to the degree that you are uncomfortable or the edge of the seat pan is digging into your lower thighs or your head tilts forward changing the curve of your neck.

Your Work Surface

The height to which you adjust your chair depends on the height of your work surface, the size and shape of your body, and the nature of your task. If your task involves a computer terminal and keyboard, it is best that your forearms are held at a 90 to 110 degree angle to your upper arms (see Figure 2.5). The forearms may need to be angled upward even more with tasks involving a typewriter (see Figure 2.6). The difference is easy to understand. The viewing screen of a computer terminal is usually several inches above the keyboard, so the hands and eyes can be further apart. On a typewriter, however, the printing of type on the paper is very close to the keys. If the forearms were at right angles to the upper arms, you would have to frequently lean forward to view the print. If your task involves much work with a telephone, calculator, or handwriting, the elbows or forearms should be allowed to rest on the work surface. This reduces the effects of strain on the shoulders and upper body from bearing the weight and muscle activity of the arms and hands. If you make mechanical drawings, blueprints, or other drawings and designs on a drafting table while sitting, the table should be angled toward you in such a way that you do not need to constantly

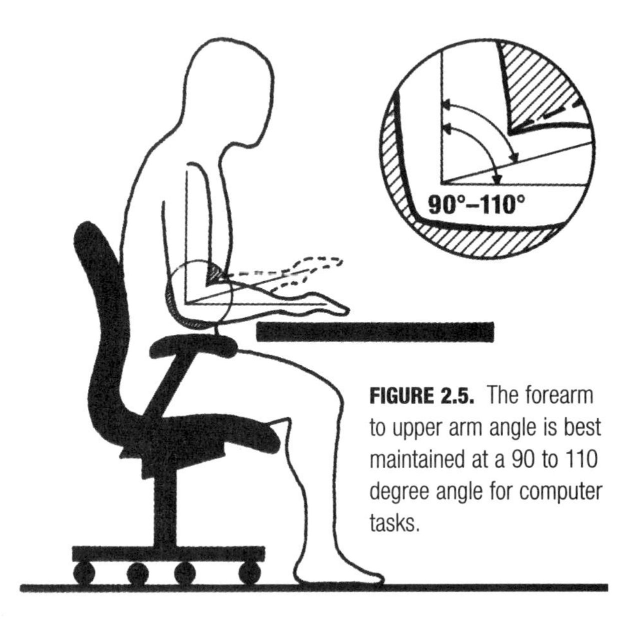

FIGURE 2.5. The forearm to upper arm angle is best maintained at a 90 to 110 degree angle for computer tasks.

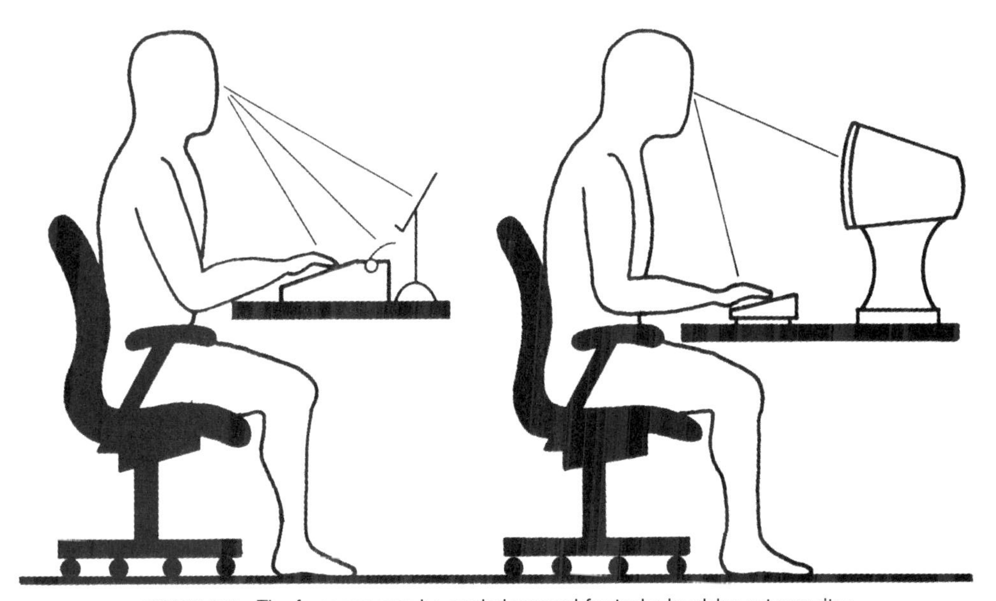

FIGURE 2.6. The forearms may be angled upward for tasks involving a typewriter.

bend your body too far forward. Tilted work surfaces are good for reading but not for handwriting tasks.

A general rule is this: the closer in distance the hands and eyes must work together for the operation of office equipment and the performance of other tasks, the higher the desk height should be (see Figure 2.7). This is to support the arms, hands, and upper body without making the body lean with the head tilted too far forward. Remember that people using a drawing board can angle the work surface toward them thereby reducing excessive forward bending.

Your task determines the proper height of your work surface in relation to your hands and eyes, as well as the angles of your arms, elbows, wrists, and hands. A work surface height and angle that could be easily adjusted would be ideal. Many work surfaces are immobile, and until recently it was not feasible to adjust them frequently. Now economical devices, such as DESKALATORS™, are available to place under the corners of your desk to raise it up to three inches. The chair height must also be adjusted in relation to the height or the work surface in order to properly fit your body.

Your chair should be angled appropriately for your comfort and your task, and the chair height adjusted so your arms, hands, and upper body fit your task. Your feet need a firm foundation to relieve pressure from the legs and to maintain your body balance. If after you have made the above changes, your legs are dangling or your feet are not firmly planted on the floor, you will need a footrest (see Figure 2.8). A good footrest should be stable enough not to shift or move about when being used, wide enough to comfortably place both feet, and have a nonskid

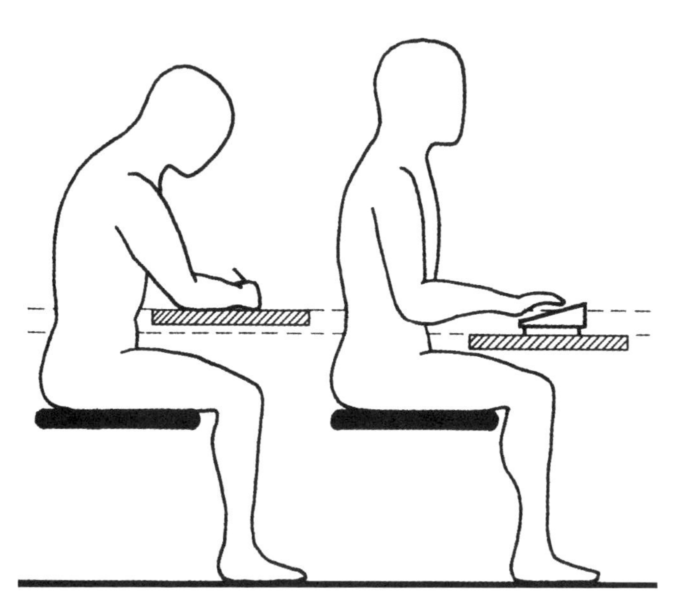

FIGURE 2.7. Handwriting and typing or keying data may require different desk heights.

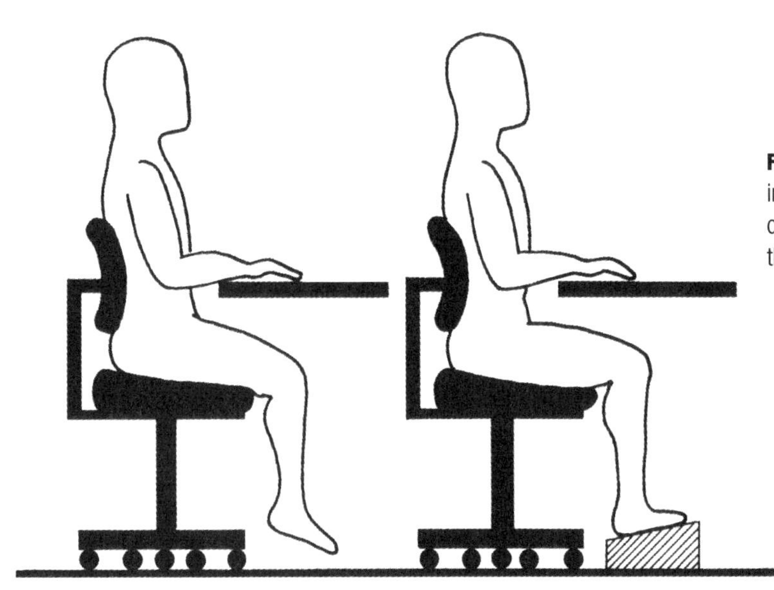

FIGURE 2.8. A footrest is indicated if the feet dangle or are not firmly placed on the floor.

surface. A footrest would be more comfortable if the surface were angled, up to 15 degrees, toward the toes. Be careful not to let the footrest restrict your leg movement and be careful not to trip or twist your ankle when leaving your workstation.

The backrest of your chair is also very important. Take advantage of it. The backrest should arch forward to support the natural forward curve of your lower spine, but it won't work unless you use it. The idea is to support the lower curve of your back to divert some of the pressure from your upper body weight into the cushion. If the cushion pushes below the waistline into the sacral bone and pelvis, it is not very useful. The backrest should fit higher to support the arch of the lower back and the spot where the forward curve of the low back changes to the backward curve of the middle back (see Figure 2.9). Support in this area will help keep the shoulders upright and reduce weight and pressure on the lower back. The only way to take full advantage of the backrest is to adjust it to fit the curve of your lower back and to make sure to sit deep in the seat so your tailbone is in the corner between the seat pan and backrest.

Some of us have short legs, and short legs mean short thighs. If this is true for you, it may be difficult to sit back far enough to take maximum advantage of the backrest without having the backs of your knees press into the chair edge

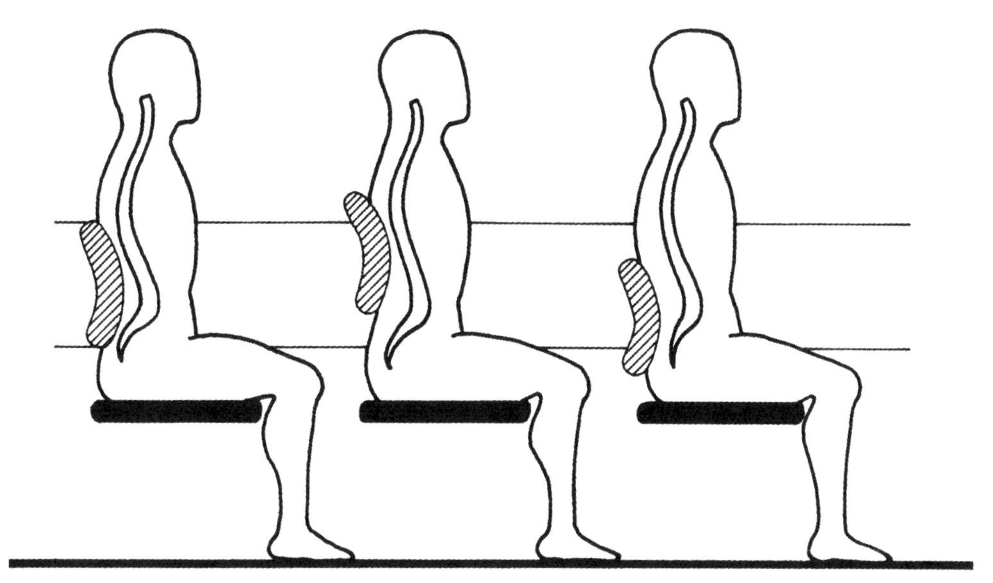

FIGURE 2.9. Proper backrest position (left). Backrest too high (center). Backrest too low (right).

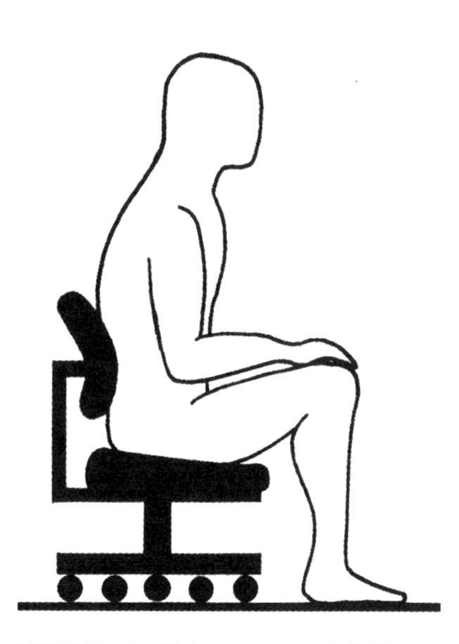

FIGURE 2.10. Make sure your chair fits your body and works for you instead of against you as in this case.

causing compression and irritation. On the other hand, if you are taller and have longer than average legs, you may feel cramped in your chair and workstation (see Figure 2.10). If either of these is your situation, do the best you can and pay special attention to the exercises and other suggestions to reduce physical stress and strain in your work. Each of us is unique in shape and size, and we need to discover our own unique physical characteristics in order to learn how to eliminate unnecessary strain from our work. The more adjustable your work environment is, the better it is for you and your productivity, but you must take the time and effort to make it conform to your special needs. Adjusting your workstation to fit you should be as important to you as selecting clothing and shoes that fit you.

A couple of additional points about your chair are important to mention. Most chairs are equipped with a capacity for rotation or swivel. If you need to turn from side to side to perform your tasks, this swivel capability is essential, but try to keep your shoulders and hips evenly aligned with each other as much as possible (see Figure 2.11). Avoid extreme twisting and leaning, especially if it involves reaching for heavy objects such as books, manuals, or catalogs. Most chairs are also equipped with four or five casters to easily move the chair from one place to another while you are still sitting. Here again, avoid twisting your body while pushing your chair from one place to another. Make sure the casters move properly and don't stick or lock at the wrong time.

For many, armrests are useful because they support the forearms, which reduces fatigue and strain on the shoulders, neck, and upper body (see Figure 2.12). Armrests also provide leverage or support to help a person get in and out of the chair. If the armrests restrict you in the performance of your tasks or are uncomfortable, they may not be practical for you. In many cases, it is simply a matter of personal preference.

Your tasks probably involve several work postures and your chair should support you in these various positions. Mr. Bill Stumpf, designer of the Herman Miller Aeron Chair and other products, used time-lapse photography to document the movements and postures of office workers during a typical day. He used this information to help him design a better chair for office workers and the results of his study were published in literature made available by Herman

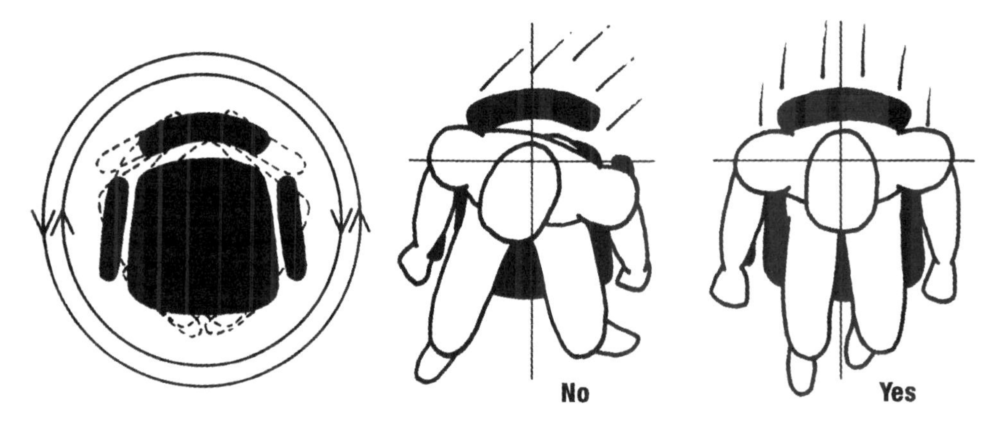

FIGURE 2.11. Use the chair's ability to swivel and roll instead of twisting and bending your body to perform your tasks.

Miller Inc. of Zeeland, Michigan, in 1982. Mr. Stumpf isolated three basic postural patterns.

First is the "work-intensive" posture. This is when you are deeply involved in a task, such as writing, typing, drawing, or assembling, and you are not consciously aware of the way you are sitting (see Figure 2.13). While in a work-intensive posture, you may tuck your legs under the chair and have a tendency to lean forward toward your work. Because you are involved in the task, the chair adjustments you made earlier are essential to allow the chair to properly support you. It is also important to develop the habit of keeping your lower back arched forward and reducing the forward tilt of your head during these activities.

Next are the "conversational" postures during which you may be reading, thinking, or talking with a coworker (see Figure 2.14). You may be frequently shifting your arms and legs or turning sideways in your chair. This posture provides you with some movement, but care should be taken to be sure your chair is still supporting your body.

Finally are the "relaxation" or "stretching" postures. When you are intensely concentrating on your task, your body probably does not move very much.

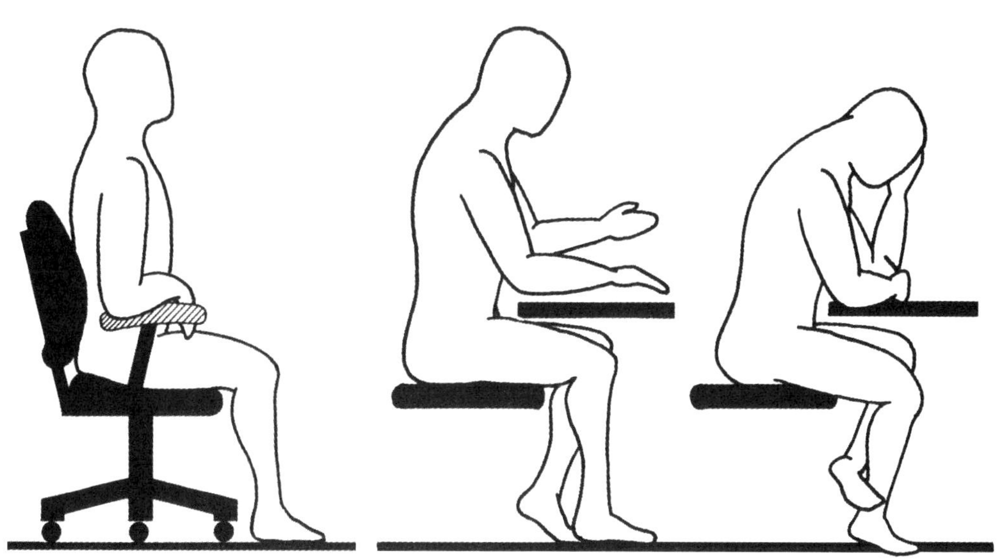

FIGURE 2.12. Armrests may help reduce muscle strain and fatigue.

FIGURE 2.13. Work-intensive postures.

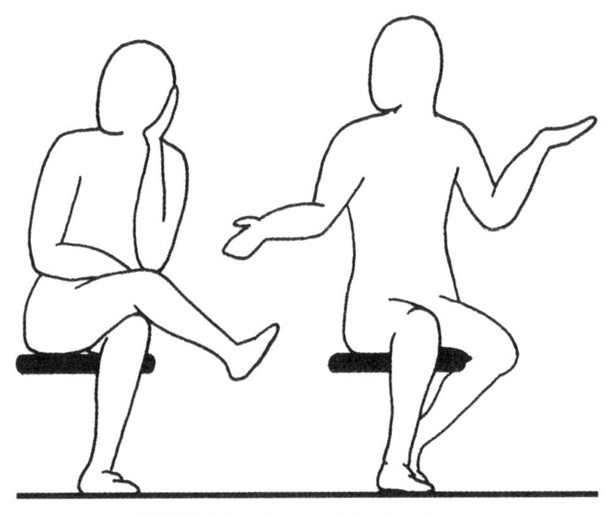

FIGURE 2.14. Conversational postures.

The buildup of tension from this stationary position needs to be released throughout the day. Use the flexibility of your chair's backrest to lean back, and also take the time to stretch your hands, arms, shoulders, neck, legs, and feet (see Figure 2.15). It is in the reclining posture that you reduce the pressure and strain in the discs of your spine and your muscles. This relaxation will help to clear your mind so you will be refreshed and ready to continue your work. You may choose to stand up and walk around for a moment or two after a period of concentrated "work-intensive" posture to help relieve your physical tension.

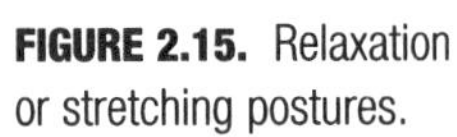

FIGURE 2.15. Relaxation or stretching postures.

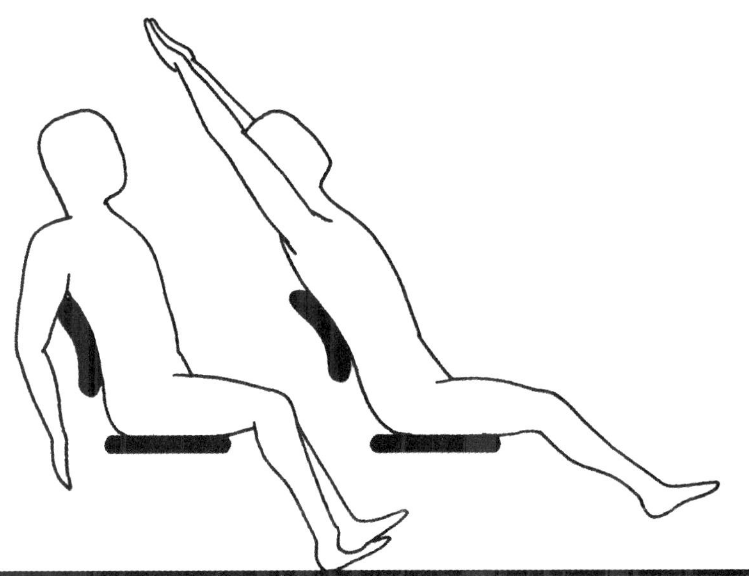

Arrangement of Work Materials

We already discussed your work surface height and some of the characteristics of your tasks involving such things as computer terminals, typewriters, telephones, and others. We will talk about each of these office instruments later, but what is important here is the arrangement of the various materials on your work surface. Let's use the airline pilot's cockpit as an illustration. The pilot sits in his or her seat with the most important item, the view of the outside world, as the main focus. The essential instruments and dials are also directly in front of the pilot, arranged around the window within easy reach. Headphones and microphones are provided to transmit and receive verbal information. Auxiliary gauges and dials are arranged around and beside the more essential instruments. Ideally, all the vital instruments are almost at his or her fingertips. Less essential controls are strategically placed within easy reach according to importance and frequency of use. The pilot does not have to twist or bend out of the seat to operate the aircraft.

Visualize this perspective in your personal workstation. The items you use most often should be placed within easy view or access, so you will not have to excessively twist or bend your body while using these items. Excessive reaching takes time and in the sitting position can strain your body, especially if it is more in one direction than the other. You should arrange the materials at your workstation in their order of priority to help reduce repetitious or prolonged one-sided movements. The nature of your task determines the arrangement of the instruments, tools, and materials at your workstation.

Computerized Workstations

Virtually every work setting involving the use of video display terminals is unique for several reasons. Work surface heights and depths vary. Workstations vary according to location in the room and create different light environments from windows, doors, and task and overhead fixtures. Our bodies vary in size and shape, so the way in which we would properly fit into a particular workstation differs. Video display terminals vary in screen size and shape, according to different manufacturers' specifications and requirements of the tasks performed. Even the size, shape, and color of the characters on the displays vary. For these reasons, in addition to your unique vision characteristics, it is impossible to give you an exact eye-to-screen distance. A generous range would be fourteen to thirty inches, but the proper eye-to-screen distance should take into consideration your visual acuity and allow you to easily see all of the characters on your video display screen without making you lean your head and body forward or backward. The characters should be clear and free from visible flickering. You should be able to hold your head in a normal posture and just move your eyes to see the characters at the extreme locations on the screen. One commonly used rule of screen position is to position the screen so that the center is at about the same level as your chin (see Figure 2.16). This could be a problem if the display screen and keyboard cannot be separated. Most video display terminal users prefer screens that are tilted toward their eyes.

If your task involves high-frequency data entry activities in which you key information from hard copy (text or papers) into a computer with a video display screen, and you only use the computer screen to check your work, the keyboard should be placed directly in front of you with the hard copy positioned on a stand also in front of you (see Figure 2.17). The video display can be positioned to the side and angled toward your visual field so you can check your work. The mouse should be positioned at the same level as the keyboard in order to minimize arm reaching.

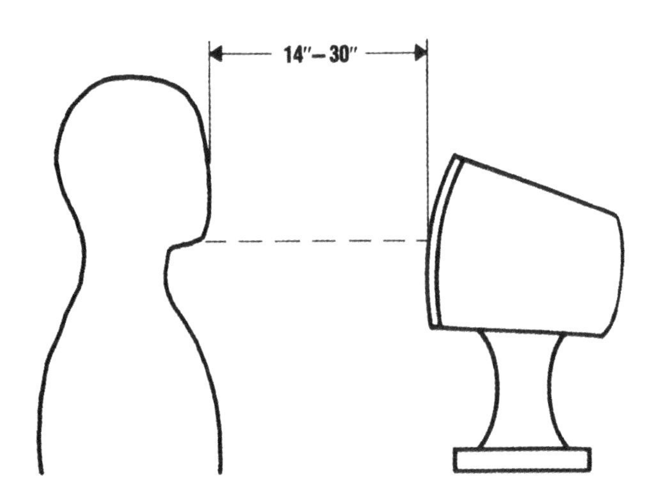

FIGURE 2.16. The eye-to-screen distance may vary from fourteen to thirty inches and the center of the screen may be most comfortable placed at about chin level.

If you have a task in which you key information into the computer to get information on the screen, and you occasionally write down some of this information, you should have the keyboard and display screen directly in front of you with paper and pencil to one side within easy reach (see Figure 2.18). Be sure to leave enough space on your work surface to allow you to write comfortably and legibly.

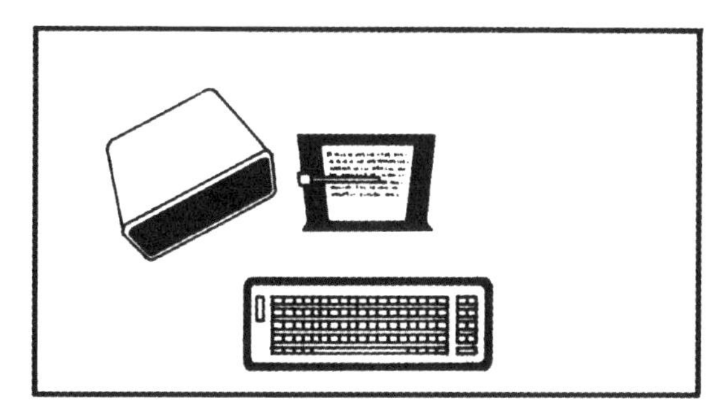

FIGURE 2.17. High-frequency data entry tasks.

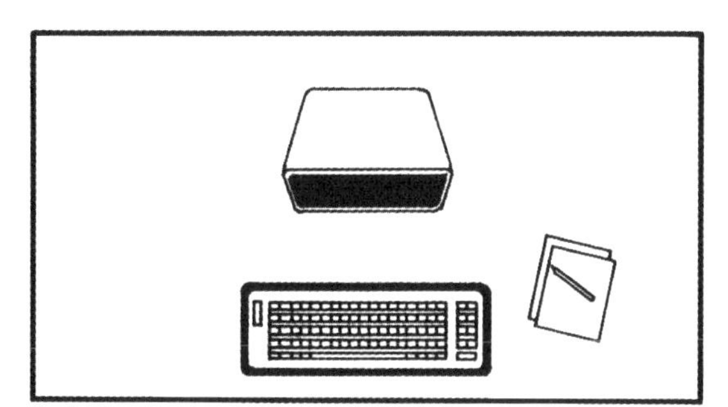

FIGURE 2.18. Retrieving and manipulating information on the screen to be written down occasionally.

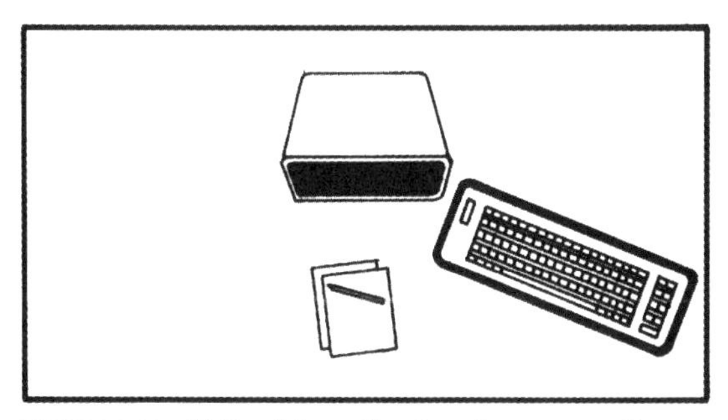

FIGURE 2.19. Writing information from the screen with occasional use of the keyboard.

If you usually write down information from the display screen and occasionally use the keyboard, the screen and your writing materials should be directly in front of you with the keyboard conveniently placed to one side (see Figure 2.19). The screen should be appropriately angled toward your field of vision.

Heavy catalogs and books should be arranged close by on the work surface in a manner that you do not have to lift or pull them with your body in an awkward position. If you need to get a heavy volume that is not within easy reach, stand up to get it or roll your chair closer to it before attempting to lift it. Whatever you do, try to prevent excessive reaching and straining.

Noncomputerized Workstations

Those of you who do not use a computer terminal with keyboard also need to arrange your workstation in order of priority. A typist usually functions best with the typewriter in front and the source document held on a stand directly above the typewriter (see Figure 2.20) or positioned closely to one side. Remember, if you constantly type with your head and neck turned to one side, you need to regularly stretch and exercise your neck and upper body to the opposite side. This will reduce or avoid restrictions with resultant spinal, muscular, and ligamentous imbalances that are accompanied by fatigue, pain, stiffness, and loss of function. You may be able to alternate the position of your hard copy from the right side to the left every few days to help reduce the effects of one-sided activities and unbalanced postures.

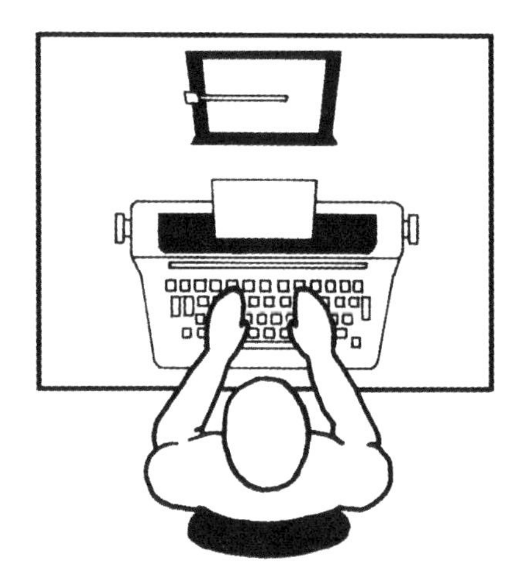

FIGURE 2.20. Typing from a source document.

You may have a telephone at your workstation. It should be positioned on your work surface according to how frequently you use it. Keep it within reasonable reach and if you talk on the phone while you are writing, typing, or keying information, avoid bracing the receiver between your ear and shoulder (see Figure 2.21). This position forces the head and neck to tilt and the shoulder muscles to be held in tension, causing strain and pressure to the neck and upper back vertebrae, muscles, ligaments, and sensitive nerves. Excessive or prolonged misuse of this posture causes neck and shoulder strain with pain and or numbness into the arms and hands as well as the potential for headaches. The conventional telephone receiver was designed to be handheld, and if you use your shoulder and neck to support the receiver, it is not being properly used. Various attachments have been designed to allow you to use the receiver in a more appropriate manner. Your local telephone, office supply, or electronics company may have several solutions available. Headphones with microphone or speaker attachments are available for those who have high-frequency telephone duties. Be sure to take the time to learn any precautions regarding their long-term use that may

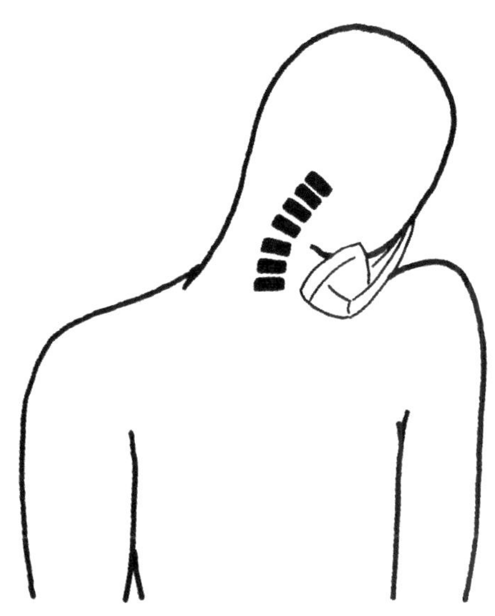

FIGURE 2.21. Bracing a telephone between your head and shoulder can cause neck problems.

affect your sense of hearing. This information should be available from the dealer representing the manufacturer of the device.

Many tasks involve the use of calculators, adding machines, and other items of office equipment not mentioned, but which may be essential to your office tasks. Use the rule of priority and frequency of use when positioning them at your workstation (see Figure 2.22). Take time during the appropriate breaks to relax, move, and stretch those parts of your body that are restricted or tensed while performing your tasks.

To operate your workstation efficiently, it is important to avoid unnecessary clutter. Everything on your desk, shelves, and in your drawers should be important to your task. Everything should have a place and should be returned to its place after use. Clutter can hide important papers and messages, and make you less efficient in the performance of your duties. Clutter can also cause stress. Take the time now to organize your workstation, using the above guidelines of priority and frequency of use. Once this is accomplished, you will feel better and it will be easier to approach your workstation at the beginning of each shift. Once organized, you must maintain that freedom from clutter. Mark down on your calendar one day each month as your "check workstation day."

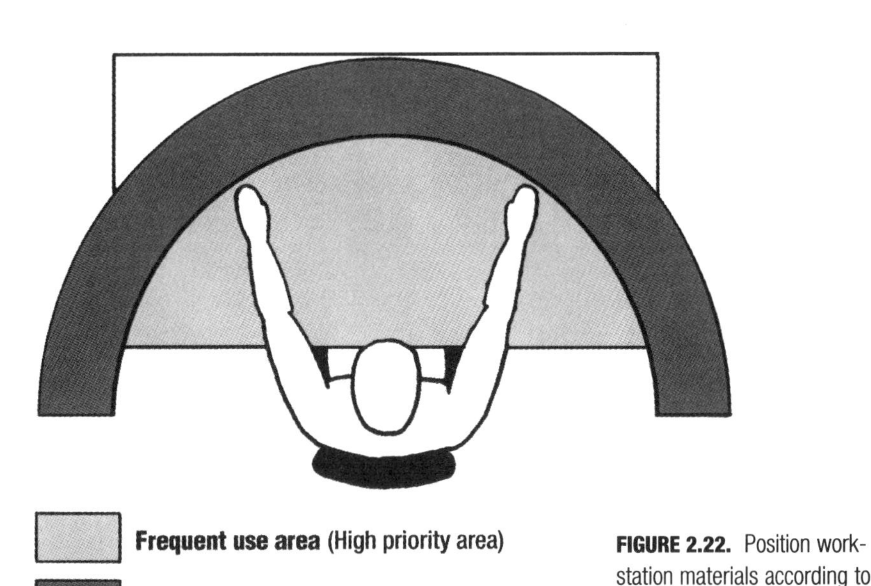

FIGURE 2.22. Position workstation materials according to priority and frequency of use.

Now you have the basics for adjusting your workstation to suit you and your unique body characteristics. It takes some work, but remember that you will be rewarded for your efforts in terms of less strain, greater comfort, and improved productivity and job satisfaction.

The Video Display Terminal

Let's face it. We are riding the wave of the computer and information revolution. John Naisbitt, author of the best-selling book *Megatrends,* has documented the course and magnitude of this wave. One of the most important aspects of this revolution is the progress and refinement of the computer with the video display terminal (VDT). The VDT has many names such as CRT (cathode ray tube), VDU (video display unit), terminal, screen, and so forth. The explosive transition into a computer world has caused a great deal of apprehension and stress in many of our lives. Fear is born of the unknown or of misunderstanding, and our fears and anxieties cannot turn back the wave of this transition. To survive and thrive, we must adapt to the present and be prepared to understand and adapt to the changes that are yet to come. If you have a basic understanding of how the computer works, it may be easier for you to adjust to the "Information Age" we have entered.

Let's examine a computer from the user's viewpoint. The video display terminal has a keyboard, which functions as a typewriter with letters, numbers, and symbols that we recognize. We "communicate" with the computer by keying the proper letters, numbers, or symbols into the central processing unit (CPU) or "brains" of the computer; it searches its memory according to the way its current program was designed to ultimately put the information we want on the display screen. The challenge is to enter commands in the exact language that the computer understands in order to get the information you need. We can also enter data to be stored for future use. This is an oversimplification, of course, but this is essentially what the computer does. It will only perform the functions for which it is programmed. It will only perform in relation to our understanding of the computer and its particular program. It was built as a timesaver and helper to humankind.

To become a successful and effective computer user, you will need to understand how to tell the computer what functions you want it to perform. When you first sit in front of a computer terminal and keyboard, it may be disturbing to you. This is a normal reaction because it is new to you. The computer terminal is an item of office equipment much like a typewriter, but it is more complex. With a typewriter, you press a key and a symbol is printed. With a computer terminal, you press a key and a great deal of information may be displayed on the screen, or manipulated in some other way. You must understand that the computer is acting in accordance to the way it was programmed, just like the typewriter was built and programmed to respond, on a key-by-key basis.

Stress involved in working with a computer may be eased by realizing that it simply responds to your command in accordance to its program and memory. Once you realize this, and thoroughly understand how to send information to the computer in the language it understands so it can carry out your commands, you will have taken a major step toward learning to relax while operating this essential piece of office equipment.

3

Your Office Environment

Many factors in your work environment directly affect your body and your ability to focus on your tasks. When you are working at your job, it is best for you and your job performance if distractions are minimal. When you are able to focus your attention and fully concentrate on your job duties, you are operating at maximum efficiency. This allows you to work faster, and with greater accuracy and consistency. This makes you and your employer happier. It preserves your employment, and thus provides for you and your family.

With this in mind, your goal is to become more aware of factors in the work environment that can be distracting to you and how you can deal with them. This knowledge will lead to greater comfort, less stress, increased productivity, and job satisfaction.

General Lighting Considerations

Approximately 85 percent of the information you receive from your environment is gathered through your eyes. Therefore, proper lighting is high on the priority list of a good work environment. Without proper lighting, you may not be able to easily see your work. Room or special task lighting should enable you to focus your vision on your work without distraction.

If your job consists primarily of using printed, handwritten or other materials that do not involve the use of a computer terminal with a video display screen, the lighting should be bright enough that you can easily see and use your materials. Inadequate lighting makes it difficult for your eyes to focus on the materials and objects. It takes more time for the appropriate information to be deciphered by the brain and for you to perform your tasks. This extra effort can cause fatigue as well as eyestrain. As the day goes on, it becomes more difficult and tiresome for you to perform your tasks.

Room lighting in this instance should not be so bright that you have to squint your eyes. While performing your tasks, avoid having direct light from windows or lamps interfere with your field of vision (see Figure 3.1). Reflections on your desk from strong direct lighting can also interfere with your ability to see and use your work materials. The cumulative effects of continually squinting your eyes to avoid bright lights or reflections can cause or contribute to eyestrain and headaches. Subconsciously shifting your body, neck, and head to avoid bright lights or reflections can cause enough stress and strain to produce or aggravate other symptoms such as neck pain, back pain, muscle tension, and fatigue.

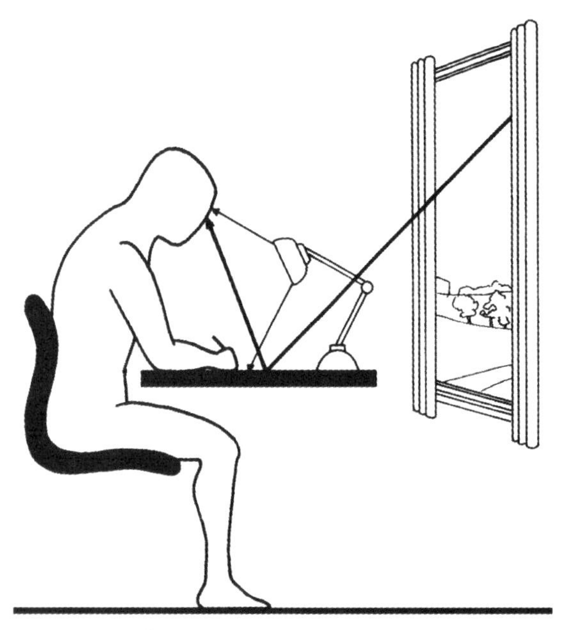

FIGURE 3.1. Direct light from windows or lamps can interfere with your vision.

Computer Terminal Lighting

A computer terminal with a video display screen combines a typewriter and a television screen with the principles of electronics and magnetics. Similar to a television screen, the VDT emits light from the screen like a flashlight. When viewing the screen from the workstation, you will notice that it has a reflective quality like a mirror (see Figure 3.2). The characteristics of lighted symbols on

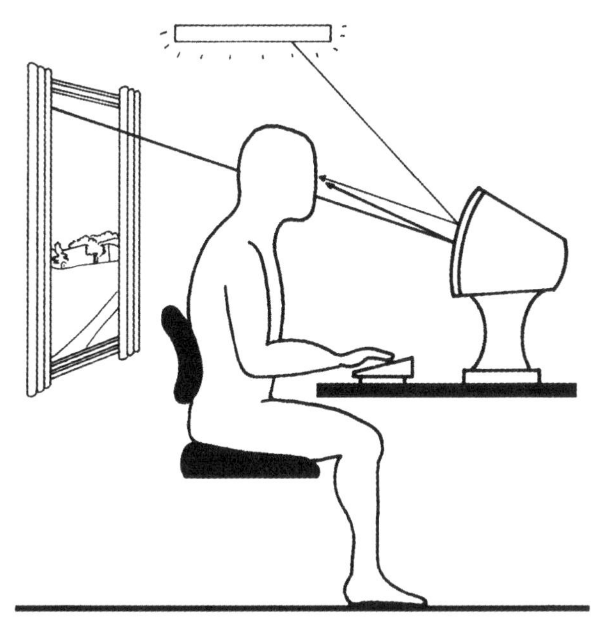

FIGURE 3.2. Reflections on a video display screen can interfere with your ability to easily see characters on the screen.

a mirrorlike screen make it difficult to place a VDT in an office that had previously been used only for typing and hard copy tasks without special considerations.

A VDT emits light, so a lower level of light is needed in this part of the workplace. In addition, the screen has a quality that reflects direct room lights into the operator's eyes causing "blind spots" to appear on the screen. A lower level of light or a different quality of overhead lighting or light fixtures may make it easier to see the numbers and characters on the screen. Even the light from windows, light-colored walls, or images from your light-colored clothing may appear as reflections on the screen and interfere with your viewing of the letters and symbols. You may have to squint your eyes or crane your neck in order to avoid the reflections or glare. These actions produce strain on your eyes, cause headaches, neck pain, or other symptoms, and can slow your work as well as reduce your accuracy and consistency. If you have to constantly work to avoid these problems, your tasks become less enjoyable.

Room Temperature and Drafts

What is considered the most comfortable room temperature varies somewhat from person to person. Some of us are more heat sensitive; others are more cold sensitive. It is difficult to set the temperature in a room with many people so that all are completely comfortable. There are, however, several things you can do to make the temperature more suitable for your body.

If you sit next to a window and the sun shines through, making you too warm (see Figure 3.3), you can pull the blinds to divert sunlight and heat.

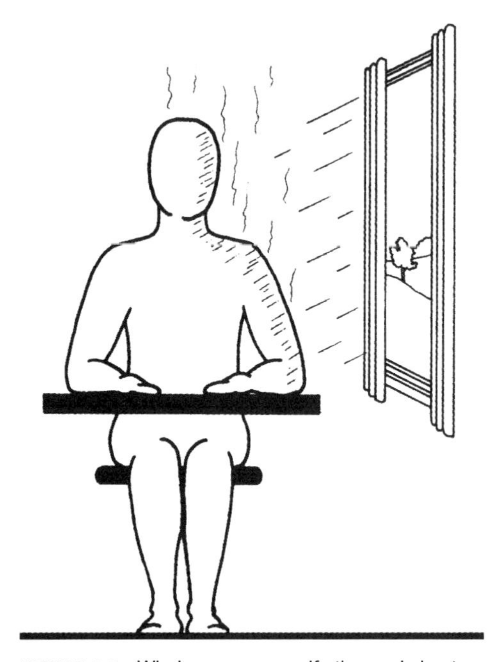

FIGURE 3.3. Windows can magnify the sun's heat and make you quite uncomfortable.

Blinds or curtains may also be pulled to prevent or reduce the chill from windows during cold weather.

Look up to the ceiling or down to the floor to locate the heat or air-conditioning vents. Forced air, whether it is warm or cool, can affect your comfort as well as your muscles. For example, if an air-conditioning vent is located above and blows cool air on you, the muscles beneath the skin that are exposed to this draft may become tense (see Figure 3.4). The tissues of your body respond to temperature changes as does the sidewalk in front of your house or apartment. When it is hot, there is expansion; when it is cold, there is contraction. If cool air blows directly on one side of your neck, those muscles will tend to become tense (see Figure 3.5). This may create muscular imbalance or tension that can pull spinal vertebrae out of alignment or create fixation, which can irritate nerves that cause or contribute to ailments such as headache, neck pain, back pain, and shoulder and arm discomfort.

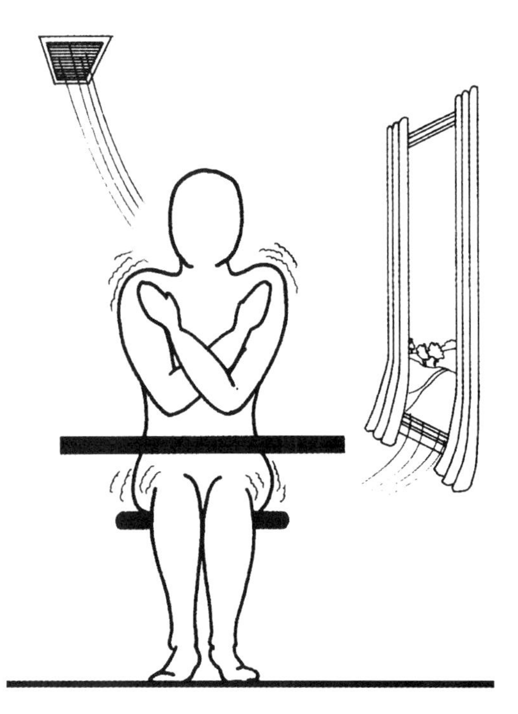

FIGURE 3.4. Air-conditioning vents can cause distracting drafts.

This reminds me of a patient I

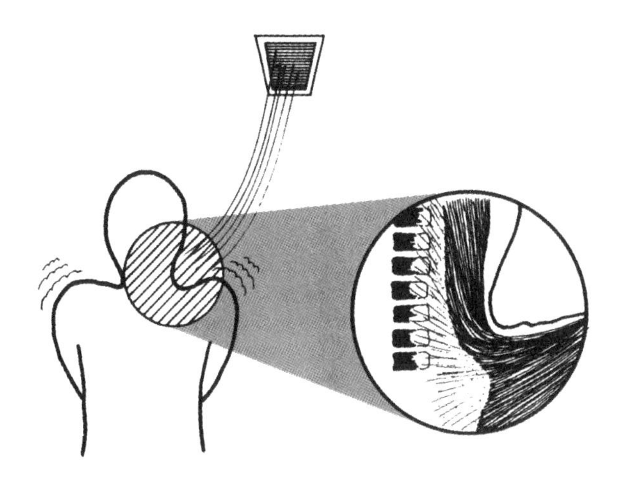

FIGURE 3.5. Cool air that blows directly on the neck increases muscle tension.

was treating for headaches. We determined that muscle tension on the right side of his neck had pulled a vertebra out of alignment, creating nerve irritation that caused the headaches. Realigning the vertebrae and relaxing the tense muscles relieved the nerve pressure that caused the headaches. He would always obtain relief from our care, but within a short period of time the headaches would return. Upon further investigation, we discovered that this individual enjoyed sleeping with the sound of a fan running. During the summer, he would place the fan on the right side of his bed and direct it to blow over his body to avoid having to run his air-conditioner. The cool breeze from the fan created muscle tension, which created a chain reaction that ultimately caused his headaches. Once he eliminated this cool draft, our treatment was successful, and he was relieved of his severe headaches.

Cool air movements and drafts can be very common, so check for these in your workplace, as well as at home. Correcting the problem may be as easy as having an air vent diverted, so it will not blow directly on your body. If you are a person who is unusually sensitive to hot or cold, it is important that you dress appropriately for the conditions you will be exposed to at your workstation.

Another important consideration in room temperature is humidity, which is the amount of moisture in the air. If the humidity is too low or too high, it can make temperatures feel warmer or cooler than they really are. Nevertheless, the effect on your body is the important factor to consider. Larry Whitehead, Ph.D., an industrial hygienist with the University of Michigan, has found that the most appropriate room environment has a humidity level between 40 and 60 percent. Some computers and office equipment require lower humidity levels, but the closer to the 40 to 60 percent range, the more comfortable most of us will feel.

Noise

Many of us are distracted by noise (see Figure 3.6). Certain noises produced by machines, air-conditioning vents, background music, and voices may distract you and interfere with your concentration. Remember, you were hired to perform certain tasks to help your business or company function, and distractions can reduce your ability to productively perform your important tasks.

Equipment noise can sometimes be reduced with proper maintenance or by contacting the equipment dealers or manufacturers to see what can be done about loud, irritating, or distracting sounds they may be producing. A telephone ring can be controlled by adjusting the volume control, usually located on the side or the bottom of the telephone. If there are many telephones in an office, the ringing can be very distracting. Be sure not to turn down the volume so low that you miss calls when you are away from your workstation. Other distracting noises and voices can be reduced with specially padded individual room dividers (see Figure 3.7), if practical and feasible. You must learn what is

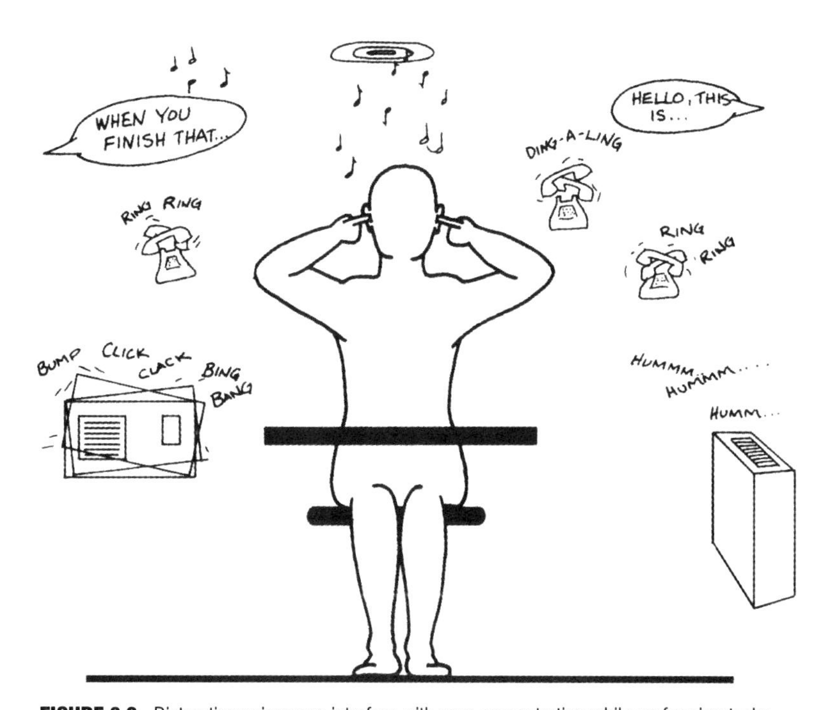

FIGURE 3.6. Distracting noises can interfere with your concentration while performing tasks.

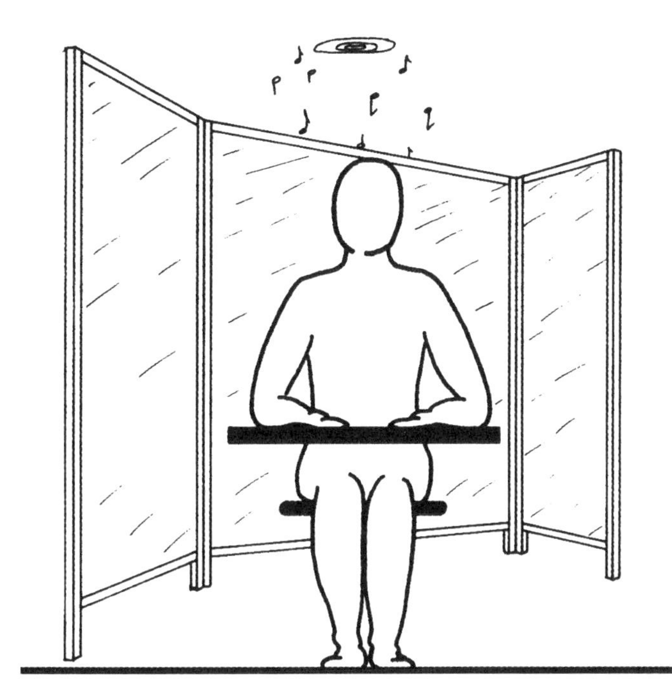

FIGURE 3.7. A possible solution to noise problems is specially padded room dividers.

most comfortable and best for you and work within that framework. Loss of hearing can also be stressful and affect your job performance, so don't hesitate to have your hearing evaluated by a competent professional if you feel this may be a problem.

You now have a better idea how you interact with your environment and some ways to detect and change your environment to suit you for greater comfort to enable you to perform your tasks more productively. We have the momentum to help carry us through the rest of this book, so let's address the common physical problems that people experience in occupations that require sitting. You'll find suggestions to help you deal with these problems, or better yet, to help you prevent them from happening to you.

4

Common Physical Complaints

Pain, restriction of movement, fatigue, and the stress these symptoms produce may be among the most prominent factors limiting productivity, accuracy, consistency, job satisfaction, and morale. Often, these factors are the reasons why many workers leave their occupations. You are not alone if you suffer from some or all of these symptoms. They are indicators of a problem, and you should do what you can to reduce or eliminate them in your life, for the consequences of suffering are too great. In addition, problems that are dealt with in early stages are usually much easier to correct than problems that are allowed to progress to a more serious state.

It is a myth that injuries and problems develop in the nerve, muscle, ligament, and skeletal systems by overexertion or improper lifting alone. Physical injuries, like sprains and strains, usually arise in one of two ways. The most commonly thought of injuries result from improper lifting, extreme physical exertion (see Figure 4.1), or from a trauma such as a fall or automobile accident. In this type of problem, a high force is exerted on the muscles, tendons, ligaments, or bones in a short period of time, causing strain, sprain, or tearing of the supportive tissues or maybe even bone fracture. Pain and swelling soon develop, and you usually know you have been injured within a short period of time.

Another mechanism for injury is when less forceful pressure is applied to parts of the body by improper movements over a longer period of time or by many repetitions (see Figure 4.2). This produces abnormal changes in the structures of the body and you may not have an immediate sprain or swelling as when experiencing a sudden, violent trauma. Pain and other symptoms of problems from these repetitious forces will develop gradually, and you may not take the appropriate actions to remedy the problems. You may not even know where or how the problem developed, unless you become educated about the way your body works and how slowly problems can develop within your body.

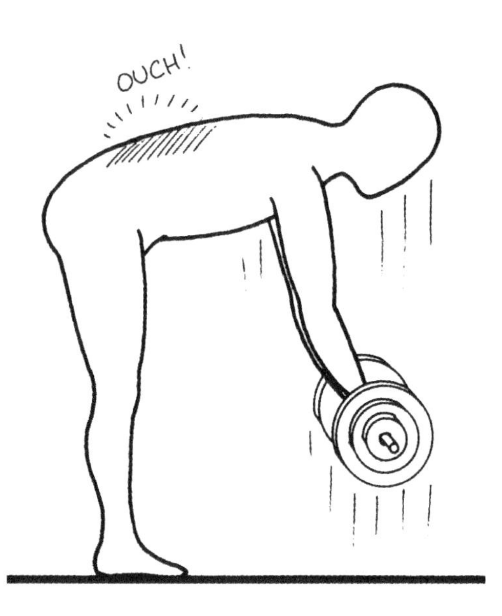

FIGURE 4.1. Injuries can be caused by improper lifting or extreme physical exertion over a short period of time.

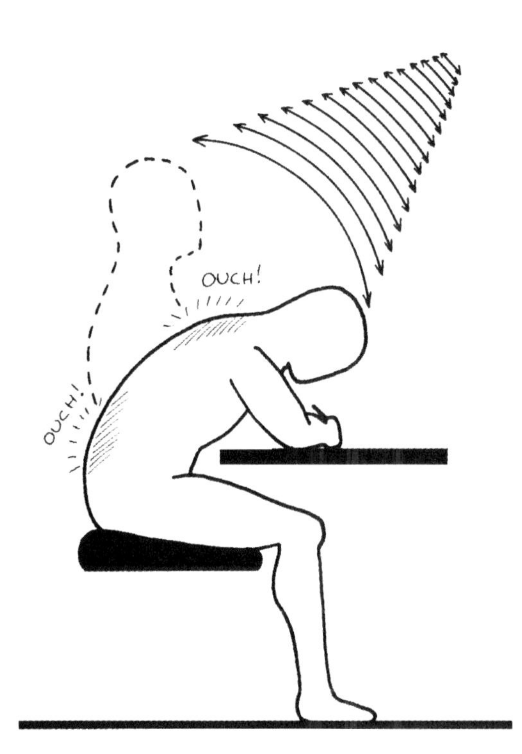

FIGURE 4.2. Physical problems can also be caused by less forceful but improper movements over a long period of time or by many repetitions.

The good news is you have already read this far. This means you care enough about yourself to want to feel better, and you care enough about your job to want to perform your tasks more effectively. Since you have already read and learned about your body and how it works, you will begin to automatically take action to investigate and remedy the problems. You have learned that sudden, excessive forces over a short period of time and slow, repetitious forces over a longer period of time can cause physical strain and sprain, which will result in painful, often disabling, symptoms.

Caution

The symptoms described here are commonly experienced among office and industrial workers and also among the general public. Suggestions described for taking action to reduce or eliminate these common complaints must not be construed as a substitute for appropriate professional care. If you have recurrent problems that are not helped by changing your workstation or using the other suggestions presented in this book, seek professional assistance. If you have questions concerning these suggestions, take your questions and this book to a qualified and trusted healthcare professional. There is no substitute for person-to-person care.

Other Causes of Physical Symptoms

One additional point before we talk about the common symptoms is that the physical complaints you may have about your work may not be singularly caused by your occupation. Previous injuries to your body may surface or be aggravated by prolonged sitting or other factors while performing office duties. For instance, if you suffered a whiplash injury from an automobile accident or if you slipped on the ice during the winter and injured your lower back, you may be much more prone to being aggravated by occupational strain (see Figure 4.3). Therefore, if you begin to experience neck pain, headaches, or low back pain, and you believe it's due to all of the sitting you are doing, you must realize that the injury you sustained several years before could still be affecting you. The pain becomes more apparent now because you are placing different stresses on your body. These problems may require professional attention in addition to applying the conservative measures suggested in this book. The same idea applies to previous shoulder, arm, hip, or leg injuries. If this is your situation, be sure to tell your doctor the full details of your previous injuries so he or she will better understand your current difficulties.

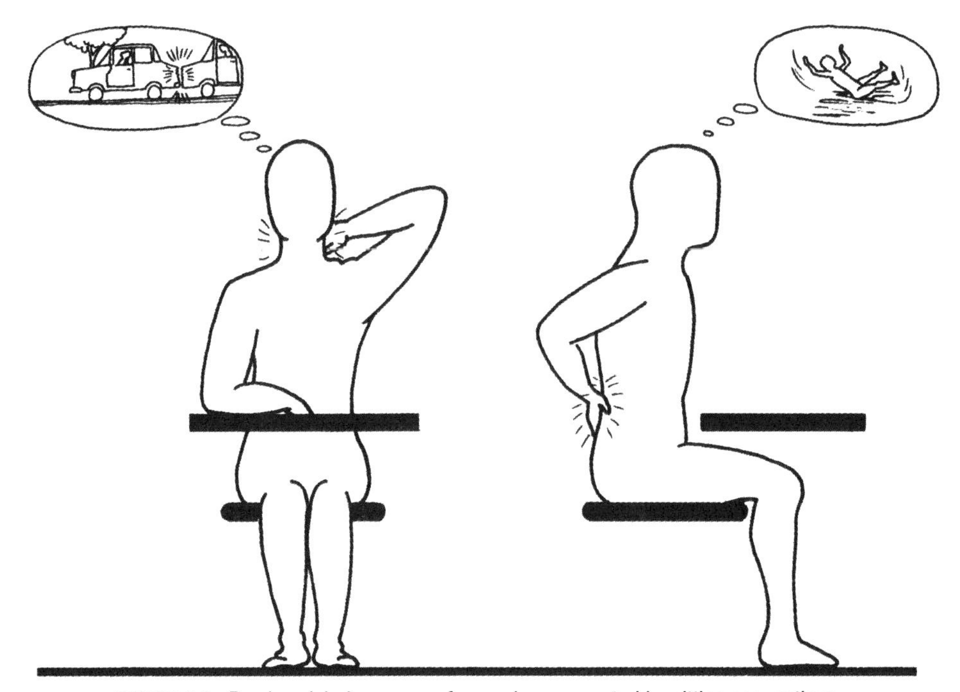

FIGURE 4.3. Previous injuries may surface or be aggravated by sitting occupations.

Eyestrain

Office and sedentary occupations usually involve a great deal of reading or studying and are therefore visually demanding. The information that I have read does not indicate that visually intensive work in itself is damaging to the retina of the eye. This kind of work does, however, pose a special challenge for the lens and for the internal and external muscles of the eyeball.

The more stress and strain you place on one part of your body, the better care you must take of that part. Most of us use our eyes almost every waking moment, and this does not cause any particular problems. If, however, you focus and concentrate on small print or objects for long periods of time, you are not using your full range of vision. The muscles that help focus the lens and hold the eye in a steady position will become strained and tired if held at one depth of focus for long periods of time, day after day. Your eyes need frequent vision breaks to minimize this strain. This means that you should frequently take a few moments to focus on an object far away. Look at the other end of the room or out the window to change your depth of vision (see Figure 4.4). This

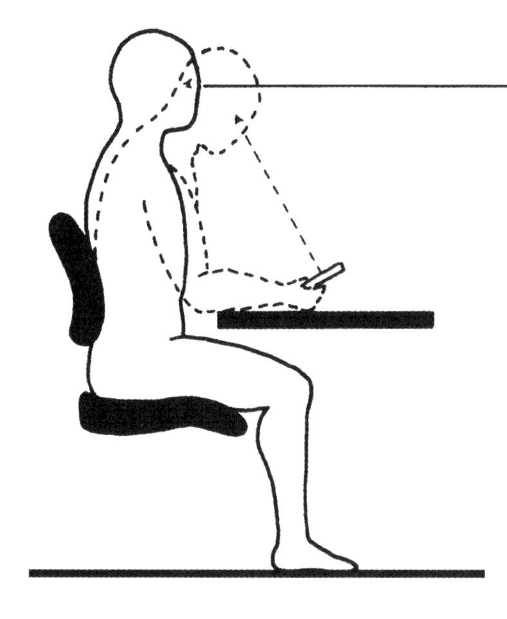

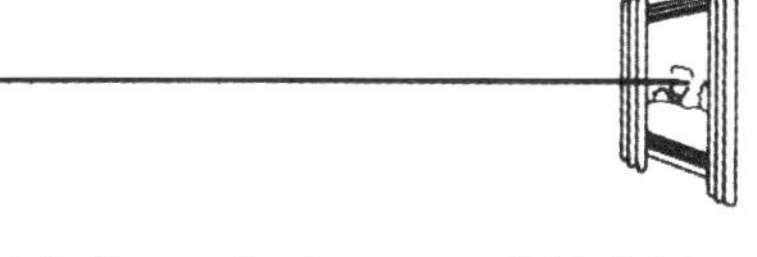

FIGURE 4.4. Frequently change your field of vision by focusing on an object far away.

also helps exercise and maintains flexibility of the lens and eye muscles. Also, take the time to roll and turn your eyes to the extremes of right and left, up and down, as well as diagonally upward and diagonally downward (see Figure 4.5). This activity exercises the muscles that turn the eyeball. These muscles obey the same rules that apply to your neck and back muscles. If you hold them in one position for a long period of time, they become fatigued. If the eyeball and lens muscles are subjected to this type of force, eyestrain develops. This interferes with your concentration and affects your job performance and well-being. Don't let that happen to you.

If you operate a video display terminal, the light-emitting characteristics, plus the reflective quality of the screen, may pose special challenges. Glare and reflection on the screen or on your desktop or walls may interfere with your ability to easily see the numbers, letters, and symbols on the screen. Under these circumstances, you may easily develop eyestrain, plus you may have to crane your neck or otherwise distort your body to avoid the glare or reflections (see Figure 4.6). This added physical effort inhibits your concentration and puts additional strain on your body. You may want to tilt or rotate the screen or

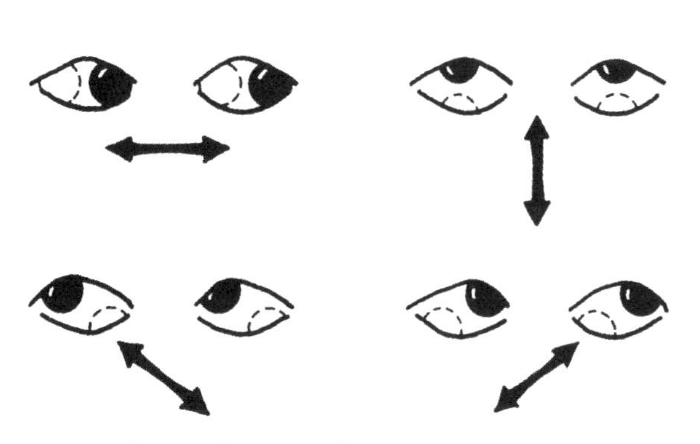

FIGURE 4.5. Frequently exercise the muscles that move the eyeball.

take steps to reduce reflections and glare at your workstation. A relatively inexpensive device, such as an Ergotron tilt-rotate pedestal base (see Figure 4.7) can make it possible for you to easily tilt and rotate the position of the screen numerous times throughout the day as light sources change. Glare-reduction screens (see Figure 4.8) are also available and helpful in many cases; however, they can be counterproductive if they interfere with the clarity of the characters on your screen.

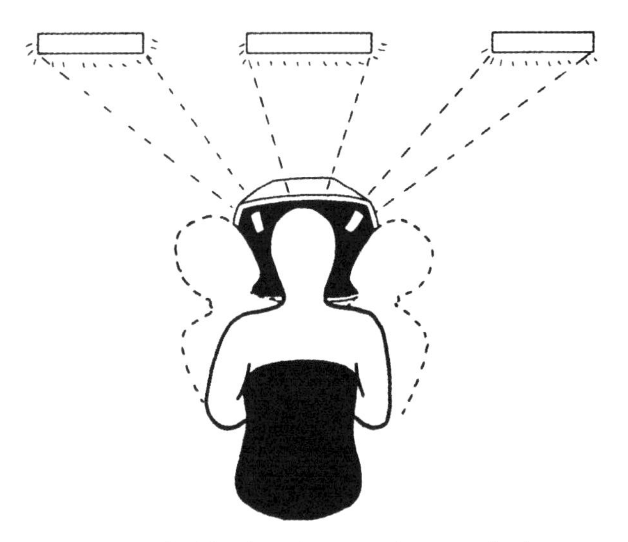

FIGURE 4.6. Looking through or around screen reflections may increase eyestrain as well as make you twist and turn your back and neck.

You may be able compensate for a small amount of excessive or inadequate lighting by adjusting the brightness control knob on your screen. This is not the ideal solution. It is best to correct the problem at the source whether it is in the light fixtures or the lights inside, windows, doors, or reflections on the screen, work surface, or walls. The brightness and contrast between the characters and the background on the screen should be adjusted so that the characters are easily read without interference.

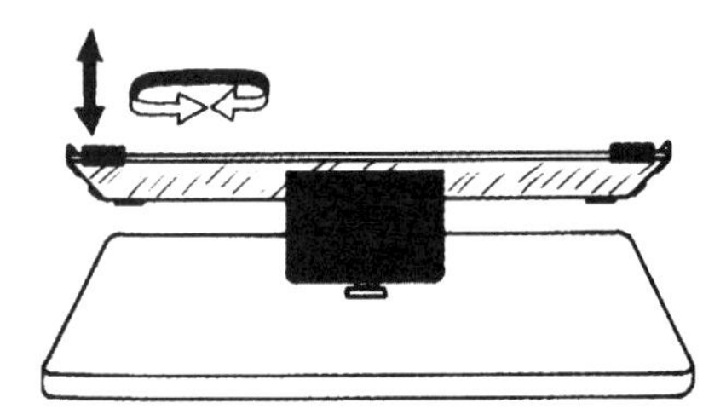

FIGURE 4.7. A tilt-rotate base on a VDT will help you position the screen to fit you and your task as well as help avoid reflections.

Flickering or unclear characters on the screen can be annoying and interfere with your concentration and comfort. These problems mean either that the brightness and contrast settings are not properly adjusted or that the VDT itself needs some maintenance.

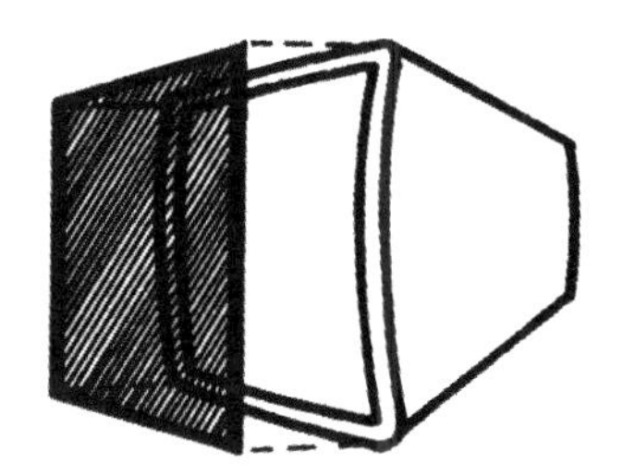

FIGURE 4.8. Glare-reduction screens can be effective against screen reflections.

Eyeglass wearers may also need to overcome special challenges. If you have bifocals or trifocals and you enter printed information into a computer, you may be looking up and down from the hard copy to the computer screen many times. This not only contributes to eyestrain, but if you have to constantly tilt your head back in order to focus on the screen, you may also develop neck, upper back, and shoulder problems and so-called tension headaches (see Figure 4.9). If this is your situation, adjustment of the height of the screen or your work surface or chair height is certainly in order. You may need to consult your eye doctor for help. Special computer glasses are available, if needed. A special coating can be applied to the glasses you use at work to reduce eyestrain arising from the special light and reflective characteristics of computer screens.

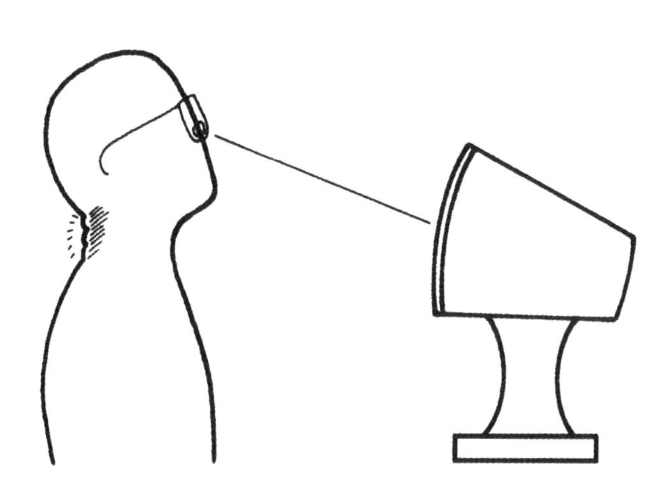

FIGURE 4.9. Tilting your head backward to view the screen through bifocals or trifocals can cause neck and upper back problems.

Back Pain

Back pain is one of the most common problems that can affect you in your work, as well as at home. It can be severe enough to make you lose time from work or annoying enough to interfere with your concentration and your ability to sit at your workstation long enough to efficiently perform your tasks. Several studies indicate that there is greater strain to the lower spine while sitting than while standing or bending. In fact, higher levels of degeneration of the bones, discs, muscles, and ligaments of the lower back have been noted in a study group of sedentary workers than in a study group of workers who handle heavy materials.

It is hard to wake up in the morning with enthusiasm if you know you are going to experience pain. This doesn't have to be the case. The purpose of this book is to help you fully understand the effects that sitting has on your back, and to provide you with information that will help you reduce unnecessary pressure and stress on your body It is important to seek professional care in cases of persistent or recurring pain.

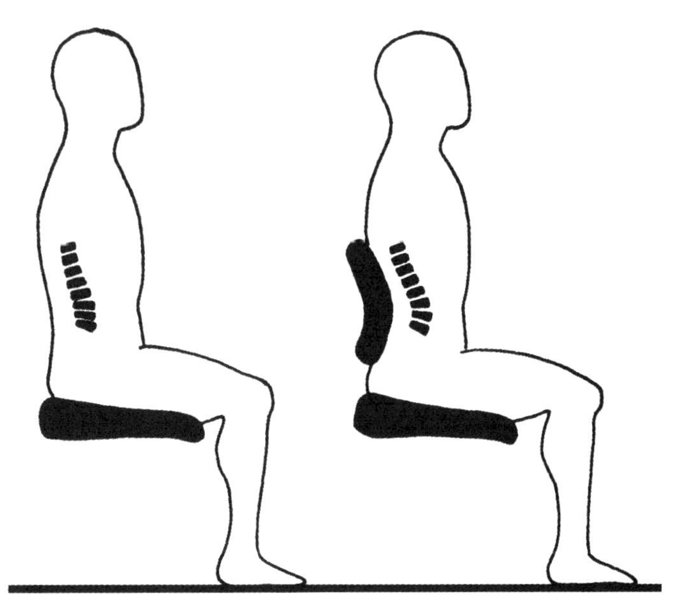

FIGURE 4.10. Unsupported sitting increases strain and fatigue. Well-supported sitting reduces strain and enhances comfort.

The main objective is to allow the chair to properly support your body while you are sitting at your job (see Figure 4.10). The idea behind a well-designed chair is for it to support the curves of the body and allow you to move into different positions as your task dictates. The chair should allow you to move, stretch, and relax your body as needed.

While you are sitting, the forward curve of your lower back should be supported at the proper position, and there should be even pressure on your sitting bones (ischial tuberosities). Your thighs should be comfortably situated on the seat pan so that the edge does not dig into your hamstring muscles. Your feet should be comfortably planted on the floor or footrest. In this position, the upper back becomes erect and your posture is good. The chair is supporting you and your spine. Slumping forward over your workstation (see Figure 4.11) takes some of the strain from the muscles, but while your lower spine bends backward, greater pressure is placed on the cushionlike discs between the vertebrae. The slumped posture creates a chain reaction that can force vertebrae out of normal alignment, producing nerve irritation and dangerous pressure on the discs. If this happens day after day, it would explain why you may be uncomfortable. If you are constantly twisting to one side of your workstation, uneven pressure is affecting your body, and the above problems will be magnified (see Figure 4.12).

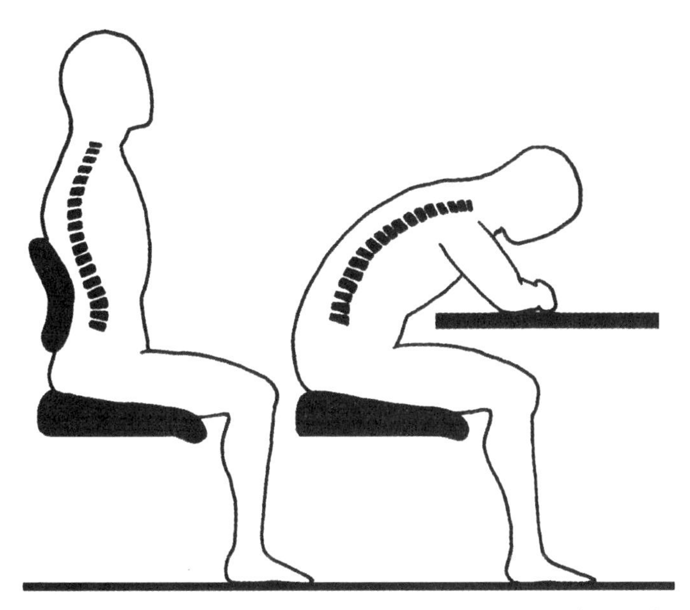

FIGURE 4.11. Using the chair's support and proper postures reduce strain and pressure on the spine. Slumping increases spinal strain and pressure.

You can see that this is a very undesirable situation, so it is very important that you make your chair work for you. It must properly fit your unique body, and you must work with it to get what you want . . . comfort and support.

Let us learn what happens to your muscles during prolonged sitting activities. Muscles are bundles of long slender cells that can contract or relax to move bones. With a steady contraction, muscles hold bones to a certain position. If you are not using your chair to help support your spine in its normal position

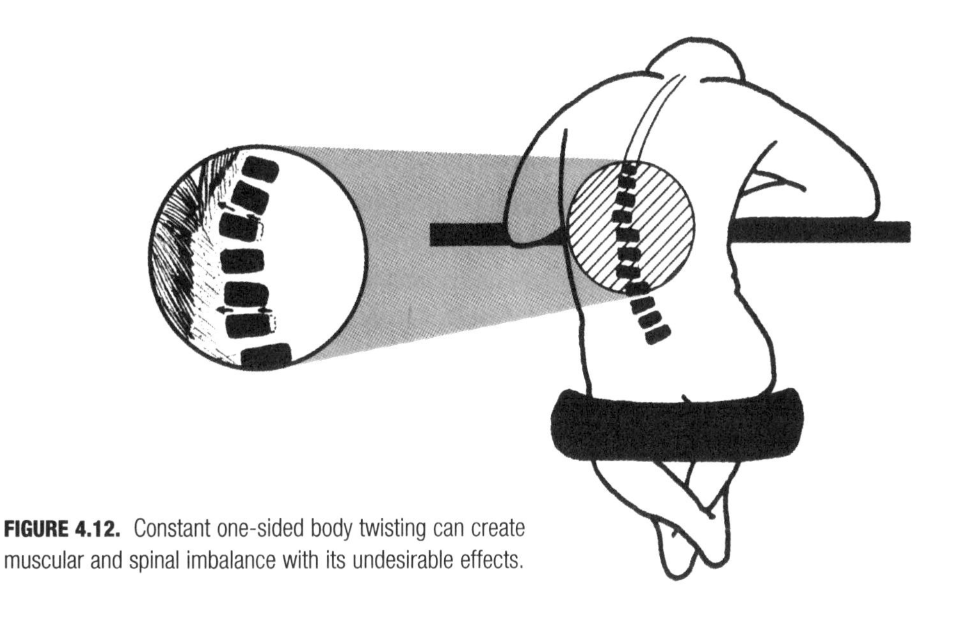

FIGURE 4.12. Constant one-sided body twisting can create muscular and spinal imbalance with its undesirable effects.

or you are not using good posture, the muscles are required to take over the load of supporting your body. When a muscle is required to maintain its contraction for prolonged periods of time, it requires extra effort, which burns more energy and creates more waste products that the body must dispose of. It is similar to the way a fire creates heat (energy), but leaves smoke and ashes (waste). The waste products of muscle contraction must be carried away by the circulatory system, but when muscles are tensed for long periods of time, the blood vessels inside are compressed so they cannot carry away all of the waste products.

Under these circumstances, the waste products—which are irritating chemicals—build up inside the muscle and make it stay tense, as well as irritate the nerves within and around the muscle. If the tense muscle is attached to the spine, it can pull and tug, creating vertebral misalignment, abnormal joint motion, pressure, and nerve irritation. Day after day, this cycle can be a major factor in the back pain you may experience. Here, again, if you must twist or continually turn one way for long periods of time or repetitiously, you may be creating imbalance between the two sides of your body, compounding your problems.

The pain and tension you suffer as the result of improper or unsupported sitting are not pleasant, but help is on the way. You have learned that you must use *your* chair to your advantage, and now you are learning that you must take the time and effort to relax and stretch those muscles that become tense. Specific exercises are explained in a section soon to follow. It is important to relax and stretch those muscles that do most of the work throughout the workday. If you take care of them, they will help to take care of you.

Neck Pain

Neck and upper back pains are almost as common as lower back pain. Though the neck does not bear the weight of the entire body as the lower back does, it holds up the head. The upper back must bear the weight of and support the shoulders and arms. A great deal of strain can be applied to these areas if precautions are not taken.

The head may weigh eight to fourteen pounds. It is supported by seven small vertebrae in the neck, which are designed to curve forward when you are looking straight forward (see Figure 4.13). But you cannot always look straight

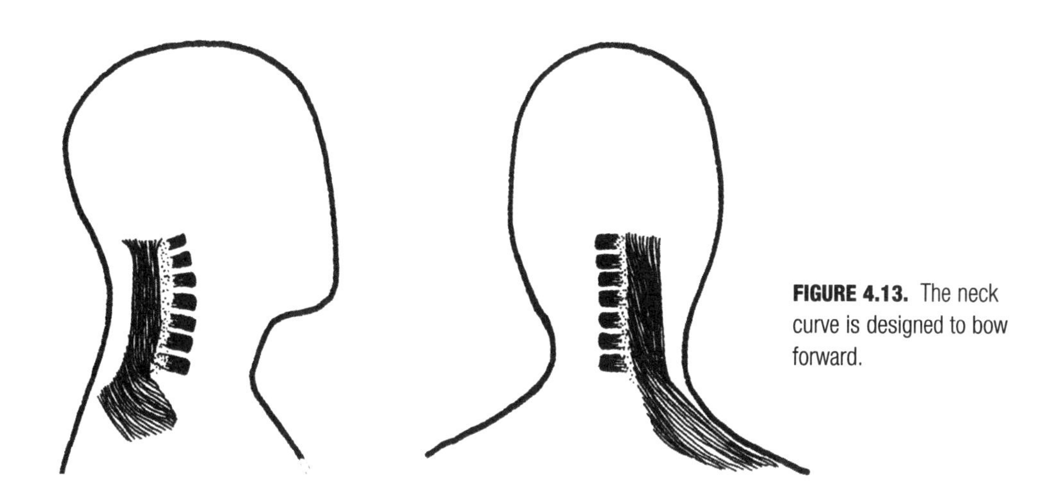

FIGURE 4.13. The neck curve is designed to bow forward.

ahead when performing your tasks. Most of the time you probably tilt your head forward toward your work surface with your chin slightly tucked to your chest. In this position, the ligaments connecting the neck vertebrae stretch on the backside and gather together in front. The muscles in the back of your neck, shoulders, and upper body tense to keep your head from falling too far toward your chest, and some of the front neck muscles tense when the head is forward. This position is within the normal range of motion for the neck and head, but if this position is held too long or too frequently without taking measures to reduce or counteract this strain, the normal forward curve of the neck can become abnormally straight or even reversed. If not counteracted, the ligaments and connective tissues of the neck vertebrae will tend to conform to the positions in which the neck and head are continually held.

Prolonged or repetitious forward head tilting or one-sided head and neck turning (see Figure 4.14) can cause extra pressure on the shock-absorbing discs between the vertebrae. Locking or fixation of one or more of the joints in the neck and irritation of the nerves that leave the spinal cord from between the vertebrae can be the result. Over a long period of time, the discs may degenerate and arthritis may develop. Nerve irritation causes pain. Nerves that leave the lower neck travel to the shoulders, arms, and hands. If these nerves are irritated at the neck, you may experience pain, stiffness, or numbness in your shoulders, arms, or hands. Nerve irritation and muscle tension at the upper neck and base of the skull may also cause headaches.

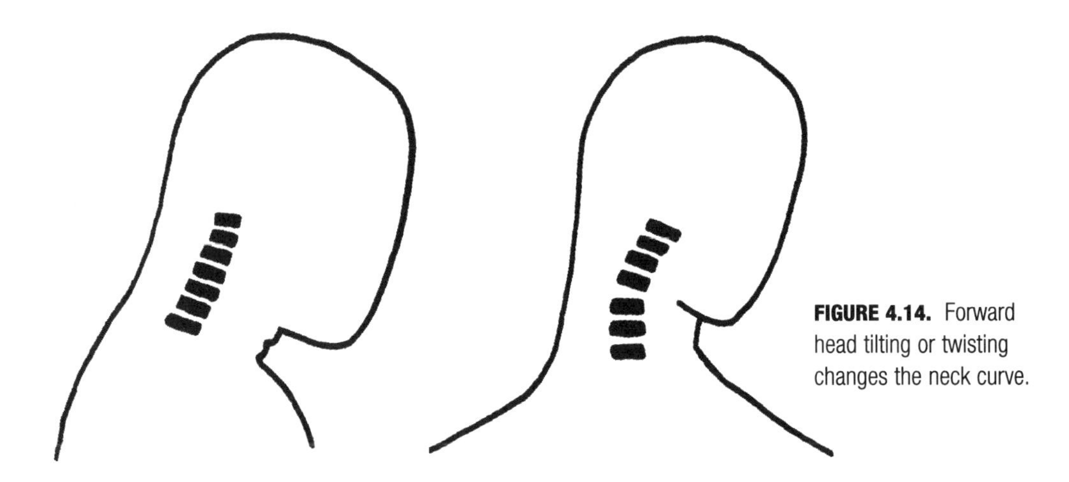

FIGURE 4.14. Forward head tilting or twisting changes the neck curve.

I know that you must tilt your head forward to some extent when you perform your tasks at your workstation, but this does not necessarily have to cause problems. It will be to your benefit to take the time to move and exercise your neck, shoulders, arms, and upper back during the workday, and take special time before and after work to counteract the effects of your particular occupation. You can also better understand how important it is to adjust your workstation and chair to fit your body and thereby reduce strain. Pay particular attention to the chapters on stress and exercise.

Shoulder and Arm Symptoms

The arms and shoulders are anchored to the body by muscles and ligaments that ultimately anchor to the spine. In other words, the weight of the arms and hands is held up by the bones, muscles, and ligaments of the upper back. If you hold your arms and hands in unrelaxed, unsupported, or awkward positions while performing your tasks, you may feel the effects not only in your arms and hands, but also in your neck, upper back, and even in your lower back (see Figure 4.15).

If you frequently use a computer keyboard or typewriter, it is usually better to keep your elbows relaxed and close to your body. This reduces muscle strain on the upper body. If this is not practical at your workstation, you may need to rest your elbows on an armrest, if available, or rest your forearms or wrists on the desktop. Sharp or right-angled edges on work surfaces that press into the muscles, tendons, and blood vessels of the forearms and wrists can cause problems, so you need to make sure that this is not a concern for you. Rounded or padded edges are helpful, but you should not put pressure on your forearms or wrists to bear the weight of your upper body. It is more practical and safer to adjust your workstation to fit your body, rather than trying to adjust your body to fit your workstation.

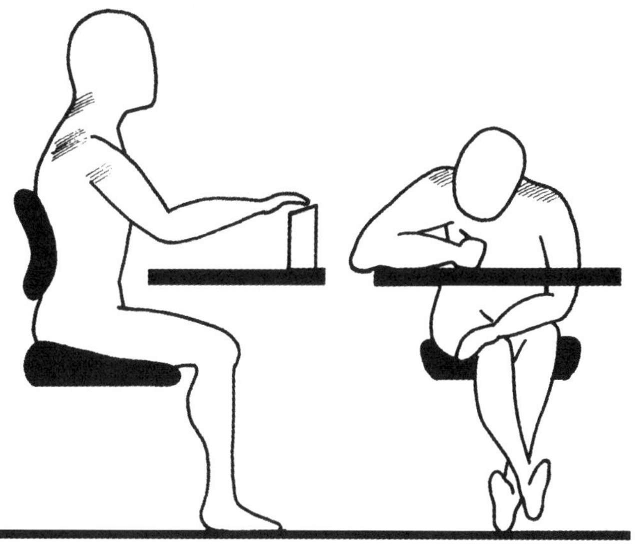

FIGURE 4.15. Arm positions and task postures can cause shoulder and back problems.

If you do much handwriting and sit with one arm and elbow spread over your work surface with the other arm at your side, your body is twisted toward your work surface. This position will become tiresome and will cause problems. Try to align your hips and chair with your shoulders to reduce the twisting and strain on your back, neck, and shoulders (see Figure 4.16). Take the necessary steps to stretch and exercise those parts of your body that become tight or strained in your work positions.

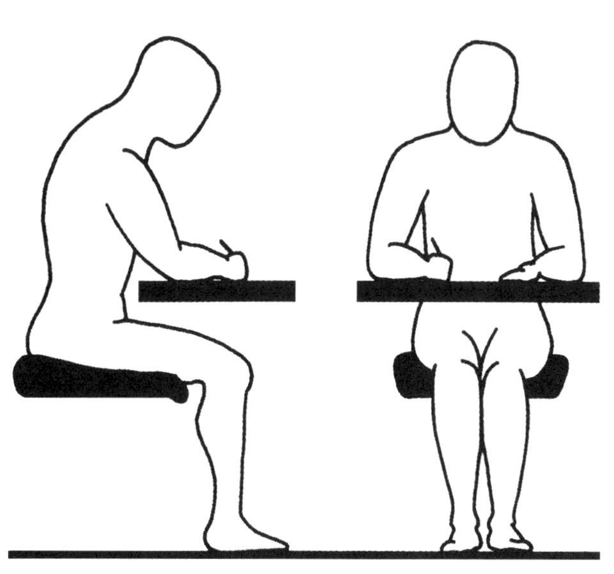

FIGURE 4.16. Align your body with your chair, your work station, and your task.

Remember, previous injuries to your neck, shoulders, back, arms, elbows, wrists, and hands may interfere with your comfort and ability to perform your tasks. If this is the case or if you have persistent problems, seek professional guidance.

Wrist, Hand, and Finger Symptoms

Wrist, hand, or finger pain, numbness, or tingling can pose a threat to your ability to perform your office tasks. Your wrists and hands are as unique as the rest of your body. In fact, if you compare your hands with those of your coworkers, you may discover that there is a notable difference in size and shape, yet you may be using the same office equipment. Proper positioning of your wrists and hands is very important in order for you to comfortably adapt to your workstation.

The wrists and hands should be used in what is known as the "neutral position" as often as possible (see Figure 4.17). In this position, the wrist is not bent forward, backward, inward, or outward. Extremes in any of these positions can put strain on the joints in the wrist and put pressure on the tendons, blood vessels, and nerves passing through the wrists. These abnormal positions also place strain on the forearm muscles and the upper arms and shoulders that anchor to the upper body and neck.

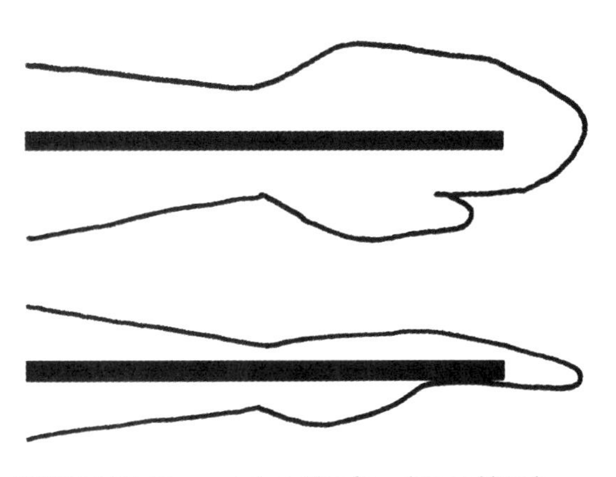

FIGURE 4.17. The neutral position for wrists and hands.

The keys on a computer keyboard, typewriter, or calculator should be positioned so that your fingers can easily and efficiently reach and press them. If you have long hands and fingers, you may feel crowded in your ability to press the keys, causing your finger joints to bend and wrists to extend toward you. You can reduce the strain of this awkward position by adjusting the keyboard to a more horizontal position (flat with the work surface) as long as it does not put your arms or shoulders in a strained position. For those of you who have short hands and fingers, a higher incline on the keyboard, typewriter, or calculator will make the keys easier to reach (see Figure 4.18). Here, again, you must

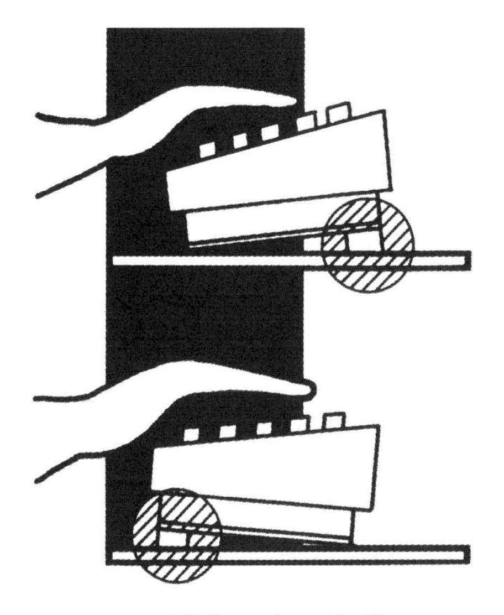

FIGURE 4.18. Tilt the keyboard to fit your hands and wrists.

be able to keep your wrists in the "neutral position" and not put strain on your forearms, upper arms, shoulders, and upper back.

If you keep your wrists and hands in a constant position while performing your tasks, it is essential for you to stretch and exercise them periodically throughout the workday and during your off-duty hours. Yes, after-work or before-work stretching exercises are to your advantage because this can reduce or counteract the effects of chronic strain. Some inflammatory and arthritic conditions make it difficult or painful to stretch and exercise these joints. Seek professional guidance if this is your case.

Make sure you flex, extend, and stretch your fingers frequently. You should also make sure your wrists get proper exercise by flexing and extending the hand at the forearm and from side to side (see Figure 4.19). The wrist does not have much motion from side to side so don't be alarmed if it feels somewhat restricted. Unaccustomed or new activities of the wrists, hands, fingers, or arms can initially result in mild discomfort. Strain, pain, or numbness that persists for more than two to three weeks suggests the need to make further adjustments to your workstation or to have these symptoms evaluated by a doctor who specializes in this type of disorder.

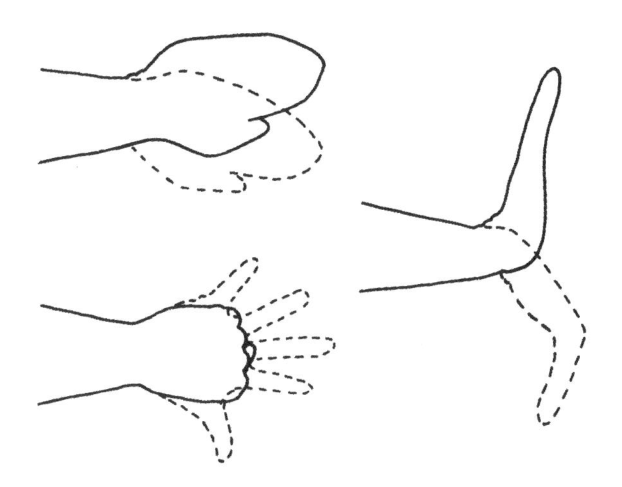

FIGURE 4.19. Normal movements of the wrists and hands.

Wrist and forearm rests are frequently used at workstations (see Figure 4.20), and they may be helpful as long

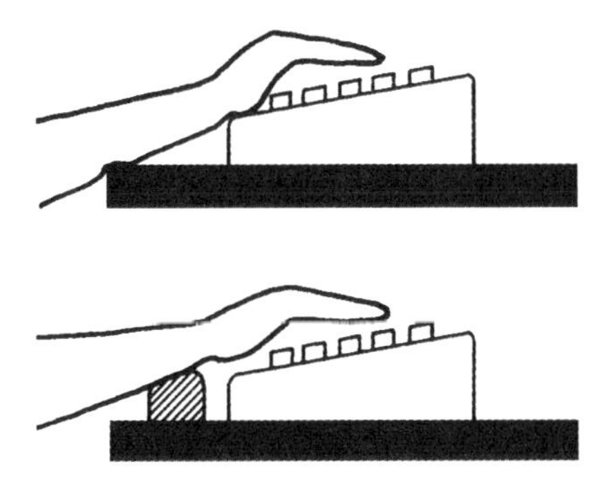

FIGURE 4.20. Avoid letting your forearms press into sharp edges of work surfaces. Wrist and forearm rests could be helpful.

as the hand, wrist, or forearm is not strained or made to bear the weight of the upper body. Be particularly careful to avoid compressing parts of the fingers, hands, wrists, forearms, elbows, or upper arms that may press into the workstation or office equipment while performing your tasks.

Some activities you enjoy during your off-duty hours can also contribute to wrist hand and finger problems. Riding a bicycle with your wrists extended or lifting weights with your elbows, wrists, hands, or shoulders in a strained positioned can aggravate symptoms you experience during work. Take a close look at your activities and postures both at work and away from work.

Leg and Foot Symptoms

Leg and foot problems may be less publicized, occurring less frequently than backaches, headaches, and fatigue, but they certainly pose a threat to your well-being (see Figure 4.21). As far as your workstation is concerned, if the chair's seat pan is raised too high for your legs so your feet are not firmly planted on the floor or footrest, there may be too much pressure on the backs of your thighs and the sitting bones of your pelvis (see Figure 4.22). This extra pressure can impede blood flow to the legs as well as stretch and irritate some of the long nerves from your spine that pass through the back of your legs to your

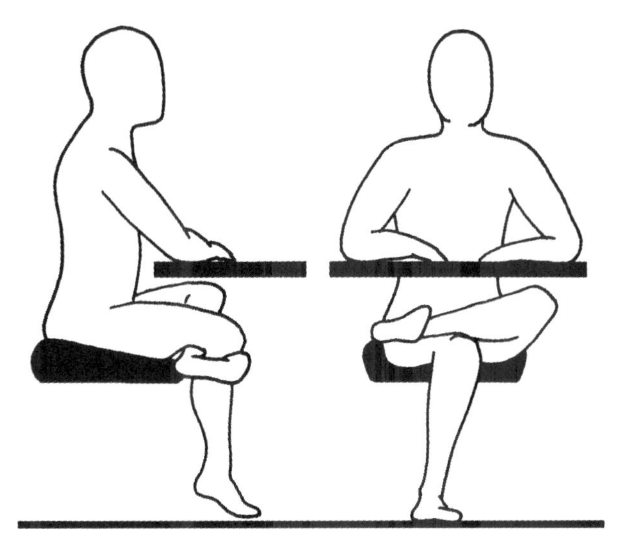

FIGURE 4.21. Improper leg and foot positions can cause or contribute to leg and foot symptoms.

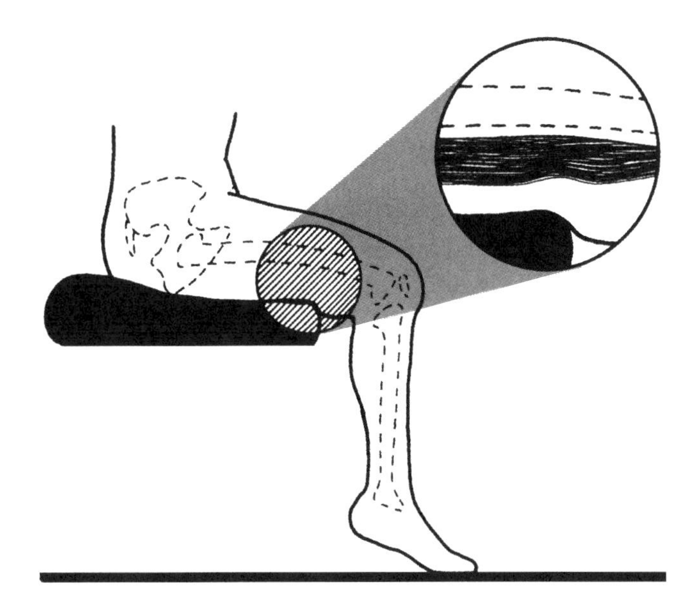

FIGURE 4.22. The seat pan angle and chair height should be adjusted to reduce pressure on the thighs from the seat pan edge.

feet. The result can be cramping, pain, or numbness in your thighs, calves, or feet. This discomfort can make you restless in your chair, and you may feel the need to squirm and twist about in an attempt to become more comfortable. This distress can interfere with your concentration.

Your chair height should help fit your body to your work surface. If it doesn't, it may be forcing you to lean toward or away from the desk. You can help compensate for this by tilting the seat pan forward or backward according to your task as was discussed in Chapter 2. A well-designed chair has a seat pan with a rounded front edge to reduce thigh pressure. The angle of the seat pan should allow the long bones of the thighs to be parallel with the seat pan.

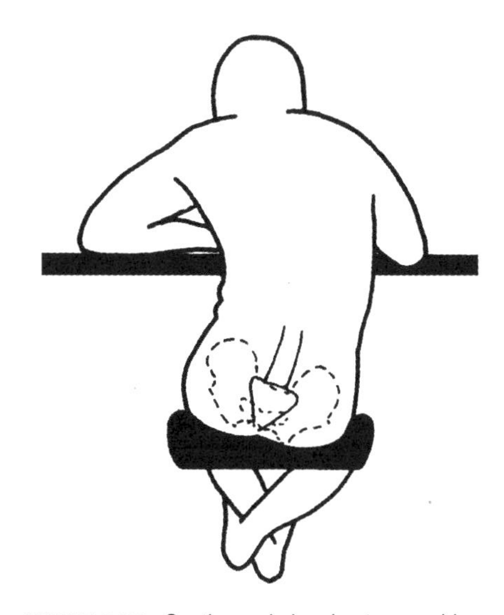

FIGURE 4.23. Continuously leaning to one side can cause excessive pressure on hips and legs.

Excessive pressure on one hip or leg can be produced by continuously leaning to one side in your chair (see Figure 4.23). This abnormal posture is usually caused by the need to turn in one direction excessively to perform your tasks on your work surface. It is important to arrange your desk, materials, and equipment so you can sit in a comfortable, balanced posture.

If you carry a billfold or notepad in your back pocket, extra pressure can be applied to that hip or leg and can crowd nerves, create muscle imbalance, reduce blood circulation, and tip your pelvis so that it becomes tilted to twisted (see Figure 4.24). This distortion shifts your lower back off center, creating imbalance and extra work for the low back muscles, resulting in spinal misalignment. The thickness of your wallet, notepad, or other objects may not seem like much, but if it is in your back pocket day after day, and you sit for many hours each day, the problems will be magnified. This is especially important while riding in vehicles, because vibration compounds the problem.

The blood vessels in the legs are a long way from the heart, which is the major pump of your circulatory system. The muscles of the heart contract to force blood from the heart through the arteries so the blood can flow throughout the body and nourish all of the cells. But the heart needs help to push the blood into and back out of the legs. Muscle contractions and movement of the legs help make this circulation easier. You can see that if you sit for long hours with your thighs and buttocks pressing into the chair or with your legs wrapped together under your chair, the leg muscles cannot help your circulation. Sitting with your legs crossed at the knees or sitting with one foot tucked under your buttocks also interferes with circulation and can cause nerve irritation along with ligament, muscle, and joint strain in the lower back, hips, legs, and feet. You need to stretch

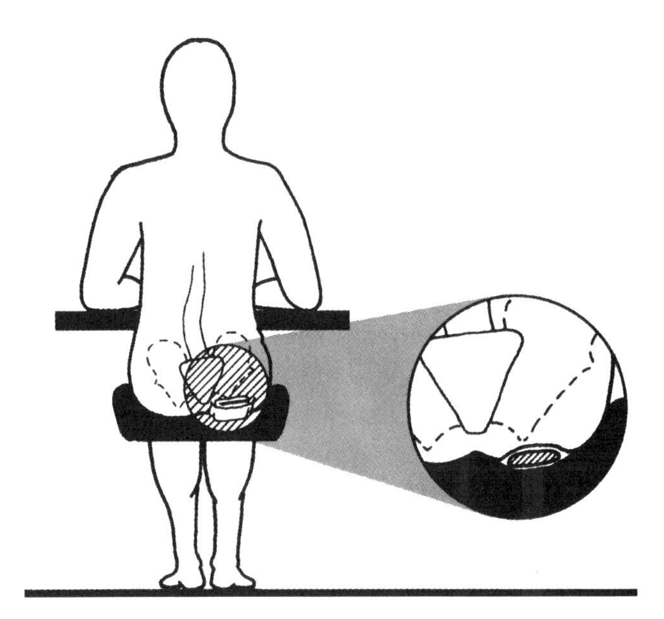

FIGURE 4.24. Billfolds or notepads in a back pocket can cause a tilt in the hips or lower back as well as interfere with circulation.

and move your legs while sitting and get up from your chair and walk about during your breaks.

Large nerves run down the entire length of your legs to the tips of your toes. These nerves come from the lower back. Nerve irritation from instability in the lower back can also cause leg, ankle, and foot problems. If you have persistent back, leg, ankle, or foot problems and you have made the necessary adjustments at your workstation and your well-designed supportive chair, you should seek professional advice to learn if a condition exists that requires correction.

Cramping, pain, or numbness in the ankles, feet, and arches can be the result of the situations described above, but can also be caused or aggravated by poorly fitting or improperly designed shoes, as well as fallen or strained arches. Well-designed and professionally fitted shoes with adequate arch supports are important, maybe not so much when you are sitting, but they become very important as you walk about during your workshift, on your way to and from work, and in leisure activities. Make sure you do not neglect this important part of your body. Problems here may not only affect your feet, but since your feet are the foundation of your body while standing, walking, and running, they can affect your legs, hips, and back.

Earlier in this book, you learned how cooler temperatures and drafts can make your muscles and ligaments contract. Hot air rises, so the coolest place in the office may be close to the floor. This cool air or the air movement from a floor vent may contribute to leg problems. Dress appropriately to keep your legs comfortable. It may be possible to redirect the air flow from a floor vent. If you know cold air is a problem for your legs, a space heater may be helpful. If you feel that you need a space heater, you must be certain you have approval from your employer, and that it is not placed in a hazardous area for you, your fellow workers, or office equipment and wiring.

Headaches

What a stressful and common problem headaches can be! In fact, 73 percent of people surveyed in a Louis Harris and Associates poll published in the October 23, 1985, issue of USA *Today* said they experienced headaches. That's almost three out of four people, so if you fall into this category, you are certainly not alone (see Figure 4.25).

There are many causes for the pain that you may feel anywhere from the base of your skull up to your temples, forehead, eyes, and cheeks. Among the causes are nerve irritation in the neck, muscle tension, high blood pressure, eyestrain, jaw joint problems, stress, sinus problems, ear problems, blood sugar problems, and the list goes on. Science has recognized about 200 separate types and causes of headaches. It is a complex health disorder requiring careful evaluation and consideration. All recurrent headaches should be evaluated by a competent healthcare provider who can perform certain tests and examinations to help you to know the probable cause and nature of your head pain. Fortunately, most headaches are not the result of a serious disease process taking place in the body.

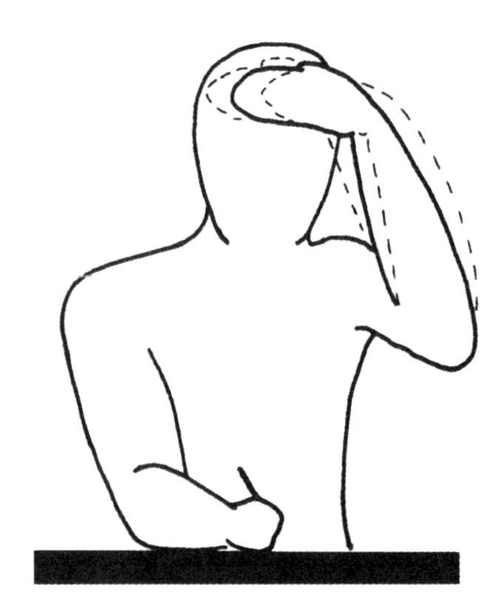

FIGURE 4.25. Headaches affect approximately three out of four people.

Let's consider how your work can cause or contribute to headaches. It is a problem to be reckoned with because headaches, like back and neck pain, can interfere with your ability to concentrate on your tasks, as well as affect the satisfaction you feel from performing your job well.

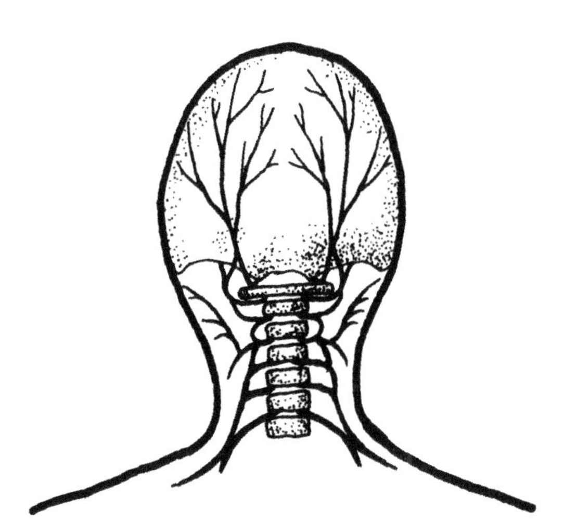

FIGURE 4.26. Nerves emitting from the neck vertebrae wrap around the skull.

First and probably foremost in office work is the complaint of the common "tension" headache. The brain resides within the skull, but most of the nerves that wrap around the head come from the base of the skull and upper neck (see Figure 4.26). The weight of your head is supported by the seven small neck vertebrae that are held together by ligaments and muscles. These muscles and ligaments are strong enough to support the head on top of the neck vertebrae, yet flexible enough to allow you to turn and rotate your head. Work postures that cause prolonged tension on the neck muscles can tug and pull on the vertebrae in a way that can create fixation or misalignment in the vertebrae, which may cause pressure and irritation of the blood vessels and nerves of the head, thus giving you pain.

Each moment that your head is away from what is called the "neutral position" (see Figure 4.27), opposing groups of neck and upper back muscles must tense or relax in an effort to hold the weight of your head within the center of gravity. If you hold your head forward with your chin toward your chest, your neck and upper back muscles are working hard to keep your head from falling too far forward, and the usual forward bend of the curve in your neck is straightened, or in some cases, reversed. Holding this position for long periods of time, day after day, without giving the strained muscles and ligaments the relaxation and movement they need, can cause the neck vertebrae to become misaligned, which creates nerve irritation and makes you feel pain (see Figure 4.28).

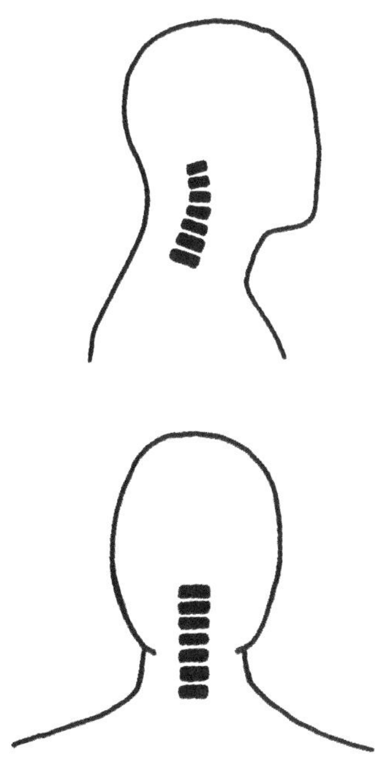

FIGURE 4.27. The neutral position for the head and neck.

If you wear bifocals or trifocals and you must tilt your head backward to see your computer terminal or typewriter, you can jam together the joints at the back of the neck, which can also result in nerve irritation that causes headaches or neck pain. Uncorrected vision problems including nearsightedness and farsightedness can make you lean forward or backward in your chair in order to focus on your work. Your sitting postures may be adversely affected causing strain and tension that result in symptoms. Office work creates a special demand on your vision, and eyestrain may be a particular problem that can cause or magnify headaches. Eyestrain and its implications were discussed earlier, but if your eyeglasses fit too tightly around your head or if they are not suited for the intensive work that you do, they should be changed. Frequent vision breaks should be taken during the course of your workday.

Turning your head to one side excessively while performing your tasks or holding a telephone receiver between your neck and your shoulder frequently or for long periods of time can also contribute to muscle fatigue, spinal misalignment, and headaches. Pay attention to how often and the length of time your head is away from a balanced and neutral position to determine if this may be a possible cause for the pain you feel.

Proper posture, chair support, workstation fit, and arrangement of work surface materials and equipment can reduce the effects that may be causing or contributing to your headaches, neck pain, or back pain.

Previous neck or head injuries, as well as problems mentioned earlier in this chapter, can cause headaches. Fitting your workstation and chair to your body and your body to your workstation, as well as exercising properly and practicing stress-management techniques can greatly reduce or eliminate your headaches. If, however, your headaches persist, don't hesitate to seek professional advice.

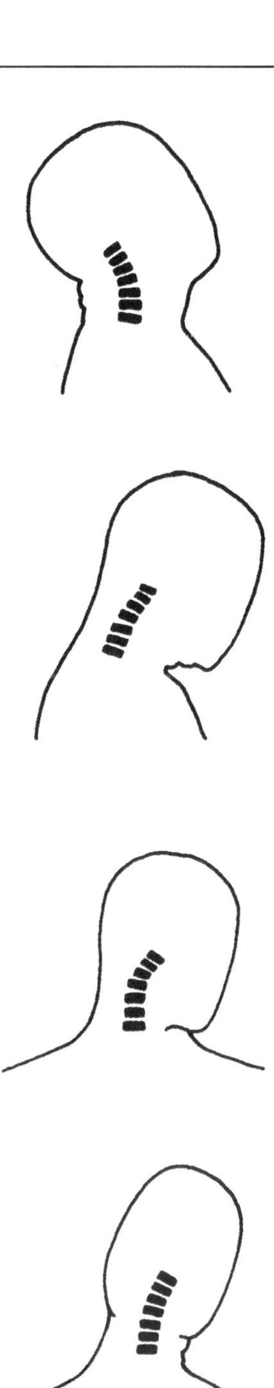

FIGURE 4.28. Changing head positions changes the neck curve.

Fatigue

Fatigue is a common complaint among workers. It is often difficult to measure, but is frequently described as a vague tiredness or feeling of low energy, lack of enthusiasm, or weakness. The major causes include the things we have been talking about: poor posture, chair support, and not properly fitting into your workstation or arranging the materials and equipment on your desk. High levels of job stress, lack of exercise, and inadequate quality of sleep and rest are also to blame. Maintaining slumped postures can make it somewhat difficult

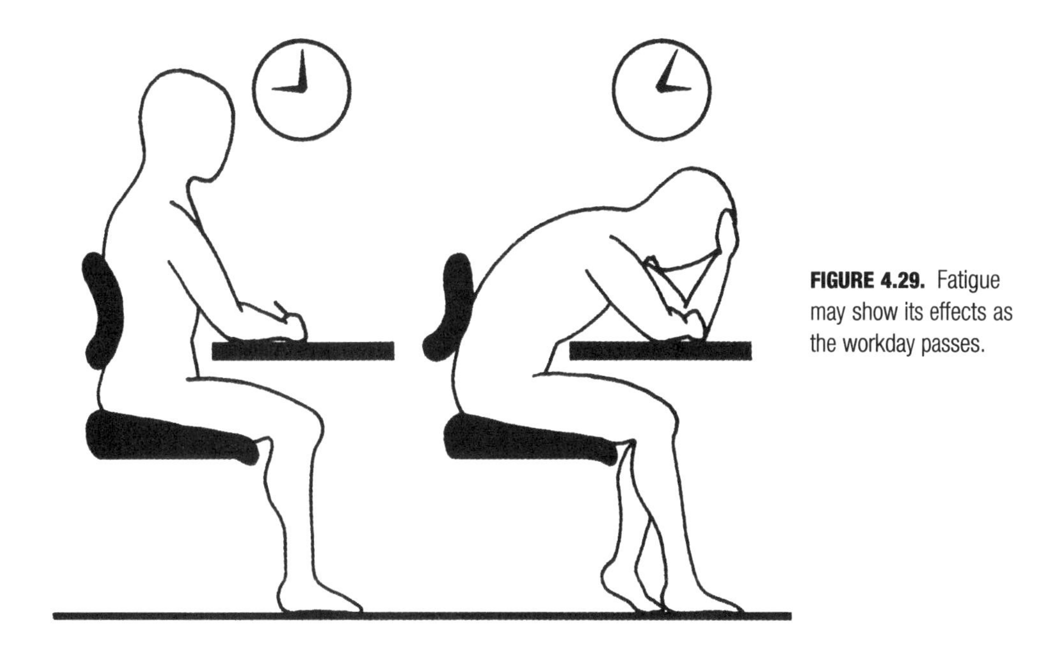

FIGURE 4.29. Fatigue may show its effects as the workday passes.

to breath in deeply and may result in shallow breathing, which also leads to fatigue.

Fatigue can demoralize you and make you acquire the attitude of "who cares if I get my work done." Your employer certainly cares about the quantity and quality of your work, and you do too, because your job depends on it. Fatigue has a quiet way of making you care less and less about your job and may even make you feel resentment for having to do your work. Attempting to live with fatigue is not the way to enjoy your work or feel that sense of accomplishment for a job done well, and it is no way to keep your present job or a possible opportunity for advancement and economic growth for you and your family. It is difficult to go to work with the feeling that you are going to be "worn out" before the end of your shift.

It doesn't have to be that way! One of the most common causes of physical and mental fatigue is lack of exercise. Yes, it may seem contrary, but you were gifted with a body that was meant to move. The body is a dynamic instrument wanting and needing exercise. Like a campfire, if you add logs to the fire, the fire grows larger and more vigorous, and if you don't add logs, the fire burns out. If you exercise your body and give it proper nutrition, your energy is preserved, but if you don't take action to keep your fire burning, it gradually goes out. This is a rough example, but it shows you how important it is to exercise and move your body. You have a special challenge that is different from a person who uses his or her entire body to perform work. You must sit in one place while performing most of your tasks so your body cannot get the exercise and movement that it needs. These special job requirements make it necessary for you to stretch and move your body during your scheduled breaks, and you should participate in work, home, or group exercise programs that will help keep your body healthy.

You now have a better understanding of how bad work postures, as well as poorly fitted or nonsupportive chairs and workstation arrangements, create strain in your body. These unnecessary strains can also be reduced by using the best possible postures and adjusting your chair and workstation to fit your body and your task.

5

Stress

Stress is such a prominent phenomenon in our lives today that you can hardly pick up a newspaper or magazine that doesn't have some reference to stress, its causes and effects on your body, or some ways to deal with the problems that arise. In fact, the mention of the word "stress" can almost create a reaction in your body. It can be such a frightful word or feeling, so let's first disarm this apparent enemy to our well-being and learn how to make it work for us instead of against us.

Understanding Stress

In the simplest terms, stress is your physical and emotional reaction to change. It sounds almost too simple, but that's what stress is: your body's reaction to change. If you perceive the change to be threatening, or you don't understand it, it can cause physical effects on your body. Your objective in this chapter is to learn how stress affects you so you can understand how to make it work for your benefit. The term "stressor" describes the situation or circumstance that causes stress (the physical and emotional reaction).

Let's say, for instance, you have a deadline to meet on the task you are performing. You say to yourself, "I have to get this done by four o'clock." Your body tenses. You know you must meet the deadline, and you focus your attention and concentrate on the task at hand, and you finish the task by four o'clock. You experience a feeling of exhilaration, pat yourself on the back for a job well done, and then relax for a while and let your body unwind.

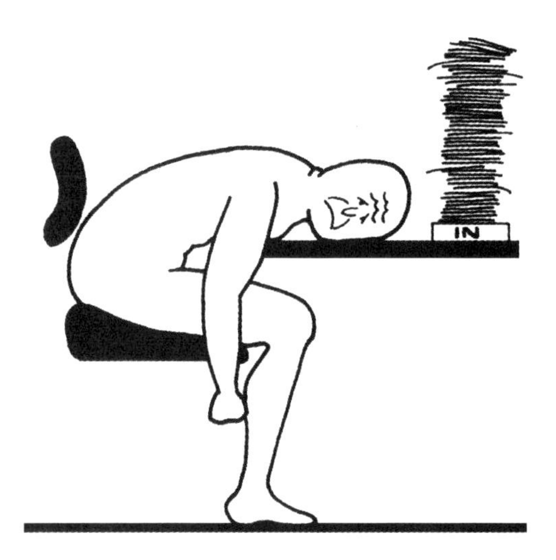

FIGURE 5.1. The cumulative effects of uncontrolled stress can make you lose enthusiasm for your work.

The stressor involved your awareness that the task had to be performed within a certain time frame. Your body and mind responded by performing the task, and then you relaxed and felt good about your accomplishment and your contribution to the operation of the company or business. During this stress cycle, certain things probably happened within your body that you may or may not have been consciously aware of. Your body geared up to accommodate the stress of the job at hand. Your muscles tensed, jaw clenched, your pulse rate increased, your blood pressure went up, your hands may have become a bit cold and clammy, and your stomach may have tensed (see Figure 5.2). These body reactions are quite normal; they are the physical reactions to stress.

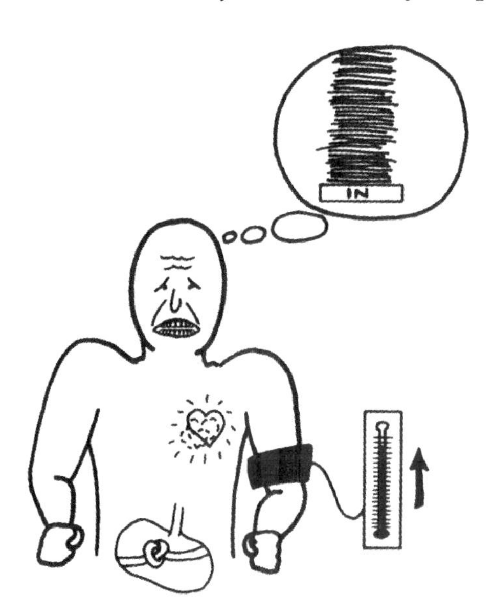

FIGURE 5.2. Physical effects of stress.

Now, suppose you perceived the stress of having to finish this particular task by four o'clock as being overwhelming, and instead of considering this to be a challenge to overcome, you feared your inability to meet the deadline or maybe even your ability to perform the task at all.

The same reaction of muscles tensing, blood pressure rising, stomach tightening, and so on would still occur, but instead of using the energy created within your body by the assignment (stressor) to focus your attention and concentrate on the task at hand, you were preoccupied with thoughts of your inability to perform the task properly or how hard the task is, to justify the possibility of not finishing the task properly or on time. With this attitude, you will probably still be tense or "stressed" even if you do meet the deadline. You may worry that your employer won't approve of or reject your work, even if it's properly completed. You may carry this heavy burden on your shoulders and, in your mind, home with you (see Figure 5.3). You may not release this stress when you go to bed, so you are still tense when you try to sleep. This can result in restless sleep, and you will still be tight when you wake up. Then, you will try to make it through the next stressful day, still carrying the weight of the previous day on your shoulders. You can see that this is a vicious cycle; it is very common, and from time to time most of us get caught in this series of events.

Congratulations are in order, because you have just jumped over the first hurdle in understanding and dealing with stress. Yes, the first step is to understand that it usually isn't stress or a stressor that is the problem. We all experience this type of pressure, but it's the way we "perceive" and the way we

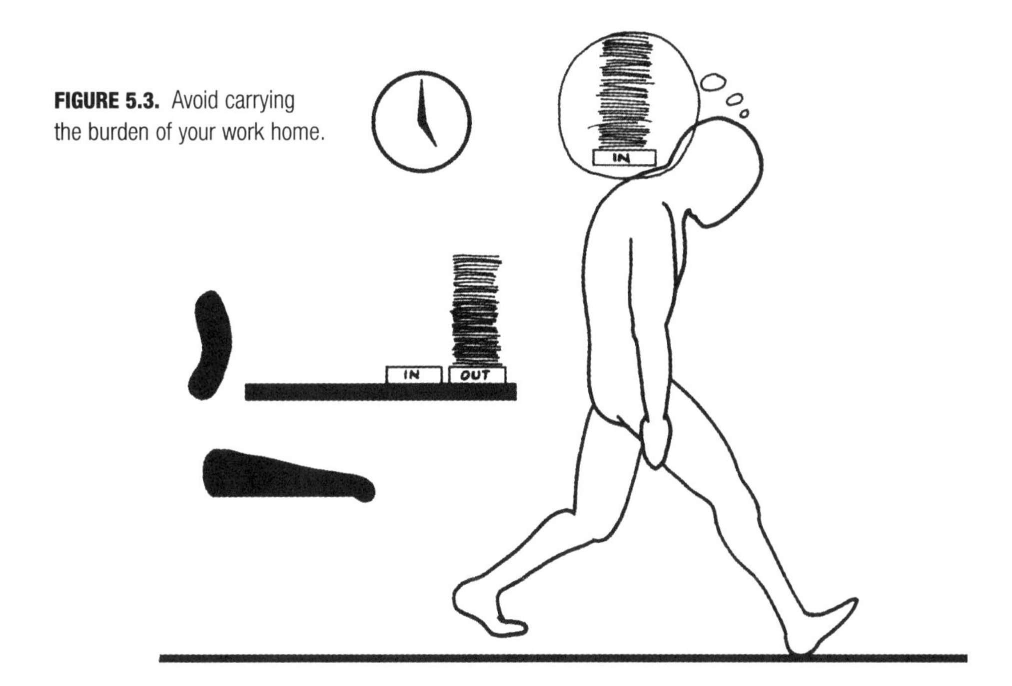

FIGURE 5.3. Avoid carrying the burden of your work home.

handle the stress or challenge that is the key. If you perceive stress to be a burden or heavy weight on your shoulders, you may question your own ability to cope, and you will get locked in to its negative effects. This drains your positive attitude and self-confidence, and robs you of the enjoyment and satisfaction you should receive from performing your job well. Remember, you were hired because your employer had confidence in you and your ability to perform tasks to help make the business prosper.

On the other hand, if you see the tasks before you as a challenge to be conquered, and you decide to take on the challenge and perform your tasks with your unique abilities, you will not only focus your attention, concentrate, and thus do better work, but you will also feel better about yourself and experience a sense of accomplishment from having successfully performed your duties.

We all know people who seem to thrive on stress. They seem to say, "Bring on the challenge! I'm ready and I will do whatever it takes to conquer the challenge in the best way I can." This sense of taking on challenges instead of being overcome by problems, combined with a feeling of commitment to conquer or succeed, can make the apparent stresses that lie before you seem fun. You can learn to enjoy the stresses and challenges that you face, not only in your work, but also in your personal and family life, by changing your attitude and the way you see your daily challenges.

Job stress creates an energy within your body that is vented, not only in physical responses, but also in your concentration of performing tasks. You need to know how to release or let go of this stress to enable you and your body to recuperate and rejuvenate so you can meet the next day's stresses and challenges with zest and vigor. Inability to vent the energy derived from meeting stress will make the physical effects of stress accumulate within your body and mind and can cause or contribute to health disorders such as emotional conditions, digestive troubles, high blood pressure, as well as causing or magnifying headaches, neck pain, or back pain.

Some say life is not a bed of roses, but I disagree. Life can be like a bed of roses! You can experience the beauty of the rosebuds and flowers, as well as the rich green leaves surrounding the bloom, but every stem grows with sharp thorns. The beauty of the rose can overpower the pain of the thorn, or the thorn can keep you from plucking the rose. Nobody floats through life without experiencing raw deals, misfortune, and sorrow, but if you are preoccupied and focus on these thorns, you will never see the beauty of the rose. It's your choice.

The healthy reaction to stress not only involves the way you perceive stress, but also the way you reverse or counteract its physical effects. The stress reaction gears you up inside, and in order to prevent this pent-up energy from accumulating in your body, you have to shift gears. This means slowing down and using relaxation or special breathing techniques, as well as engaging in some form of enjoyable physical exertion such as aerobic exercise, swimming, bicycling, racquetball, or tennis, to use up or vent the inner energy built up during periods of stress. This shifting of gears, both higher through enjoyable exercise, and lower through relaxation techniques, will help keep stress from accumulating and getting you down.

Let's look at the relaxation techniques. Many techniques exist, but some of the more common and easily used are progressive relaxation, positive imagery, deep breathing, and focusing. If you feel more comfortable about beginning stress reduction or other techniques described in this book with the help of a qualified health professional, be sure to do so.

Progressive Relaxation

Progressive relaxation was developed by Edmund Jacobsen in the early 1900s. The theory is that when we experience mental stress, we tense our muscles, and the physical discomfort of knotted muscles makes our mental stress worse. The objective here is to break the tense-mind-tense-muscle cycle (see Figure 5.4).

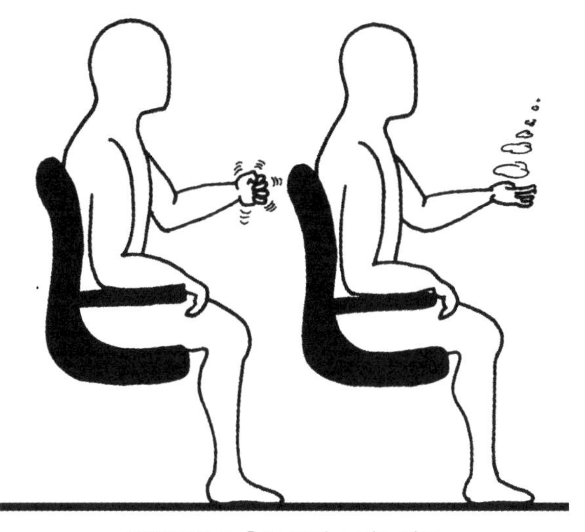

FIGURE 5.4. Progressive relaxation.

Progressive relaxation consists of alternately tensing and then relaxing different groups of muscles, forcing you to focus on how it feels to relax. Here are the simple steps:

1. Sit in a comfortable chair or lie on the floor with your feet against the wall, and close your eyes.

2. Make a tight fist with your right hand, hold it for about five seconds and experience the tension.
3. Unclench and let the tension flow out, noting how it feels different to relax.
4. Do the same with your left hand and the muscles in your upper arms and shoulders.
5. Tense your neck, hold and relax, noting the feel of the relaxed tension.
6. Frown as hard as you can and relax.
7. Smile as hard as you can and relax (remember how it feels to smile and be sure to use these muscles more than your frowning muscles).
8. Raise your toes (or push against the wall) feeling the leg tension and relax. Again notice how the tension drains away.
9. Take a deep breath, feeling the tension in your chest. Exhale and relax. Breathe in again and hold, then exhale and concentrate on how calm you are.
10. Daydream that you are in a peaceful, pleasant setting and enjoy it for a while.
11. Now count slowly to four and open your eyes You'll be fully alert and relaxed.

A daily session of this technique may take about twenty minutes, but as you practice, it can be much shorter. This technique may be impractical to perform at your workstation, but if you take the time and form the habit of using progressive relaxation daily, you will benefit, not only in your work and job satisfaction, but also in your general health and well-being. Consistent use of progressive relaxation will also make you consciously "tuned in" to your body so you can sense when tension or strain begins to develop so you can take care of it sooner rather than later when the symptoms become more severe.

Deep Breathing

Deep breathing is another simple technique used to help combat the tension buildup experienced by most office workers (see Figure 5.5). Just follow these easy steps:

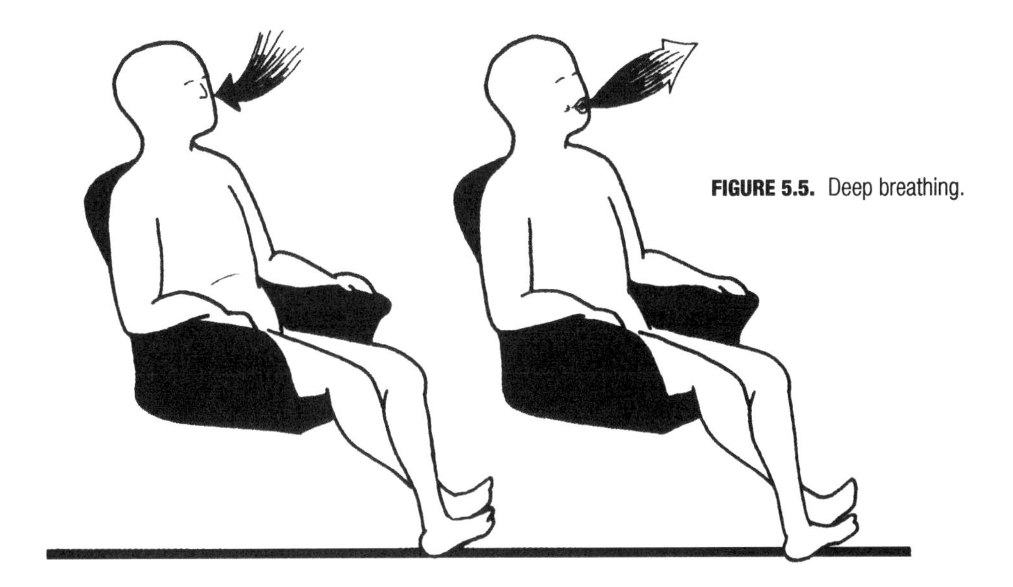

FIGURE 5.5. Deep breathing.

1. Sit in your chair or stand comfortably, but erect.
2. Place the palms of your hands against your stomach.
3. Breathe in slowly through your nose, but allow your stomach to expand forward against your hands.
4. Hold this deep breath for a few seconds.
5. Slowly exhale through your mouth, slightly pursing your lips together, and feel tension draining away.
6. When you have exhaled as much as you can, repeat the technique.

You should repeat this cycle a couple of times at the beginning and work up to taking four or five breaths in this manner after some practice. Be careful not to breathe too fast as this may cause hyperventilation or lightheadedness. If this is the case even after you have properly performed the technique, contact a health professional. This technique can also be performed during short breaks during your workday, as well as at home.

Positive Imagery

Another less time consuming, but enjoyable method of relaxing your mind is through positive imagery or controlled daydreams (see Figure 5.6). According to psychologist Jerome L. Singer, you can follow these simple steps:

1. Lean back in your chair and become as comfortable as possible.
2. Breathe in slowly through your nose and out through your mouth about ten times with your eyes closed.
3. As you breathe out, say to yourself, "calm," or "relax," or just "ommm."
4. After about two minutes, picture a positive, beautiful, and peaceful scene from your own experience and imagine yourself to be in it. Keep engrossed in the scene until you feel the tension draining from you.

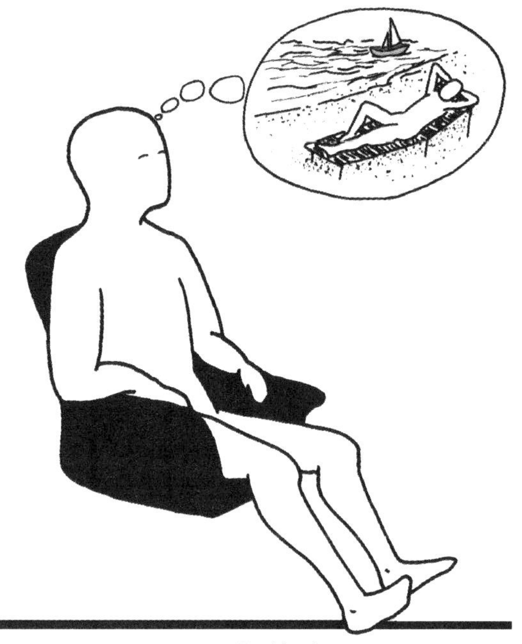

FIGURE 5.6. Positive imagery.

5. Open your eyes, arise from your chair, stretch, and you will be ready to go.

You may be able to use this technique on mini breaks during office hours, as well as at home.

Focusing

Focusing is another valuable method for identifying and dealing with stress. This technique was developed by psychologist Eugene Gendlin. This is a way of recognizing your body's signals that something is wrong, that your body is reacting to stressors with tensed muscles or gritting teeth. Take a "strain inventory" every day. Check out situations that might be stressful and that keep you from "feeling great." First, you need to recognize how stress affects your body, whether it be tense neck muscles or back muscles, headaches, or stomach aches. Once this is known, you can write down which stressors affect you and to what degree. If you write them down, you have a better chance of finding solutions to counteract the stressors' effects. By this focusing or analyzing, you can gain a sense of control over stress and find yourself in a better position to adapt to the changes you encounter.

Helpful Health-Building Practices

Chiropractic care has long been reported by its patients as an effective means of interrupting the tense-body-tense-mind cycle. Remember that when we undergo long periods of stress, the muscles become tight and tense, and can pull on the vertebrae and create fixation, restriction of motion, and resultant nerve irritation that perpetuates the cycle. Careful removal of the fixation by a licensed doctor of chiropractic interrupts this cycle and makes other stress-reduction techniques and procedures more helpful.

The concepts, philosophies, and techniques involved in practicing yoga can be an extremely effective means of relaxing to overcome the tensing effects of stress. Deep, rhythmic breathing combined with slow, controlled stretching certainly deserve careful consideration when organizing your stress-management program. There are many good books and classes available today. One is Richard Hittleman's *Introduction to Yoga.* Be sure to use proper precautions when beginning this type of program. You may need supervision or professional guidance.

The soft tissue stretching and relaxing feeling experienced by a good massage can also help to counteract the cumulative tensing effects of stress. These procedures should be administered by properly licensed and certified individuals. It may be wise to check with your doctor before entering into a program of massage.

The techniques discussed have taught you how to shift to a lower gear, to relax your body and thereby help you to counteract the effects of stress. You have also learned that you must discover what your major stressors are so you can pay particular attention to them while organizing your plan of stress management. It is essential to form the habit of practicing stress reduction daily not only to survive but also to thrive in the pressure-filled work arena, as well as in personal and family life.

Exercise

Now let's learn how to shift to a higher gear to bum up and vent some of the effects of stress. Your body produces chemicals during stress to mobilize your body in a "fight or flight" response. But you are sitting in a chair and using limited movement to perform your tasks. The muscles are tensed and your body is prepared for vigorous or quick activity that seldom takes place.

Structured physical exercise can be an extremely effective method of reducing stress (see Figure 5.7). You should plan a time to systematically vent this unanswered instinct for physical action. Researchers have learned that people under stress who work out regularly stay healthier than those who don't. Many businesses have recognized the value of exercise and have installed gyms and running tracks for the benefit of their employees.

Exercise provides a physical release of the effects of stress, and when this is accomplished, there is usually a relaxing or calming effect. Enjoyable exercise, as well as other hobbies, can provide a diversion from the stresses of the day, plus provide personal fulfillment (see Figure 5.8). Dr. Herbert A. DeVries, director of physiology at the Exercise Research Laboratory, University of California, has shown that even mild rhythmic exercise, such as regular walking or cycling, can be more effective in stress control than tranquilizers without the adverse side effects of these drugs.

Exercise is such an essential factor in stress management and general wellness that Chapter 6 is devoted to this topic. Use what you can, when you can, according to the schedule that you make. Be sure you choose exercise activities you find enjoyable and beneficial or you will feel forced to do them. This may not only cause you stress, but you may also find excuses to delay, postpone, or quit. You must regularly and consistently exercise for maximum benefit. Feel good about giving your body what it needs!

Laughter can also have tremendous therapeutic value. Laughing at jokes, at

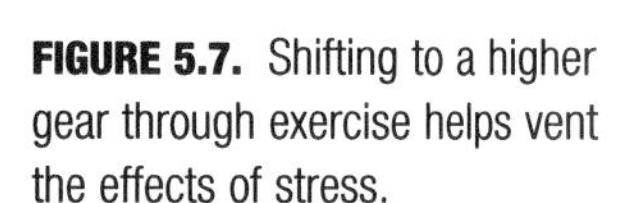

FIGURE 5.7. Shifting to a higher gear through exercise helps vent the effects of stress.

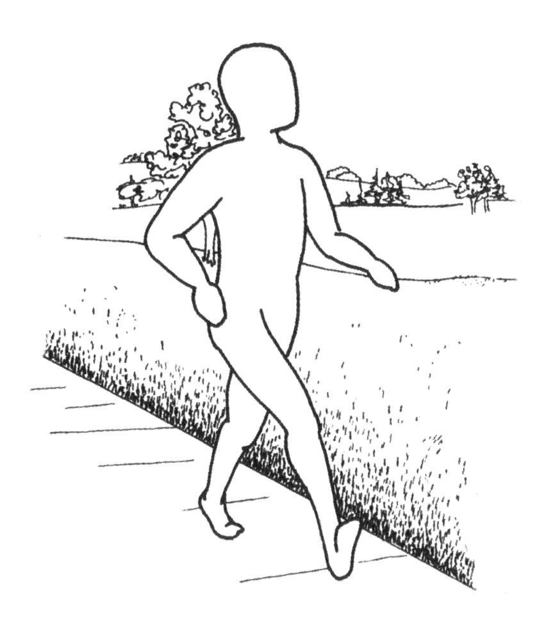

FIGURE 5.8. Enjoyable exercise can provide a diversion from daily stress.

life, and at yourself can serve to put your stresses into perspective. Laughter, like vigorous exercise, not only satisfies emotional or mental needs, but it also seems to create positive chemical changes in the body that promote health and well-being. It's bound to make you feel better. The famous author and editor Norman Cousins used laughter that he described as "internal jogging" to help cure a stressful "incurable disease." His book *Anatomy of an Illness* may provide you with some enlightening insights.

As mentioned earlier, hobbies can also provide an important diversion from stress. We live in a marvelous time in history in which we can take advantage of many pleasurable activities. Choose hobbies that you enjoy and that do not add to or compound stress on your mind or your body. Take advantage of whatever brings you pleasure, including music, movies, dancing, or any other activity that interests you, relaxes you, and refurbishes your mind.

The Stress-Resistant Person

If you want to survive and thrive in this stressful life, you will need to work to acquire the attributes and perspective of a stress-resistant person. Two stress experts, Suzanne O. Kobasa, Ph.D., and Salvatore R. Maddi, Ph.D., report in their book, *The Hardy Executive: Health Under Stress*, that individuals who were successful in coping with stress had three characteristics not found in those less hardy.

Unlike the less hardy individuals who view change as a threat to their security, the hardier individuals perceive change as a natural challenge to master. They see life as strenuous, yet exciting, and welcome change as an opportunity for improvement. They also have a strong sense of commitment to themselves, their families, their jobs, and other important values. In contrast to less hardy individuals who find tasks boring or meaningless, hardy people involve themselves zestfully and with maximum effort and interest to what they consider important missions (see Figure 5.9).

Hardy individuals exhibit a sense of optimism or control over their lives. Unlike less hardy people who see themselves as passive victims of forces beyond their control and expect the worst, hardy individuals believe they can influence events. Instead of taking a situation at face value, they try to turn a possible negative into an advantage. As Zig Ziglar, a famous motivational expert, expresses it, "Turn the lemons thrown at you in life into lemonade."

Now what's in it for you to work hard to acquire these hardy characteristics? Drs. Kobasa and Maddi have shown through their research that people who view life's stresses and change with challenge, commitment, and control are only half as likely to become ill as are the less hardy people exposed to the same stress levels. These inner resources proved to be more important and effective antistress factors than genetic makeup, relaxation methods, or exercise. What's especially exciting is that these hardy characteristics, while usually learned during childhood, can be developed. It's your choice. You can do it if you are willing to change your attitude and acquire the appropriate habits.

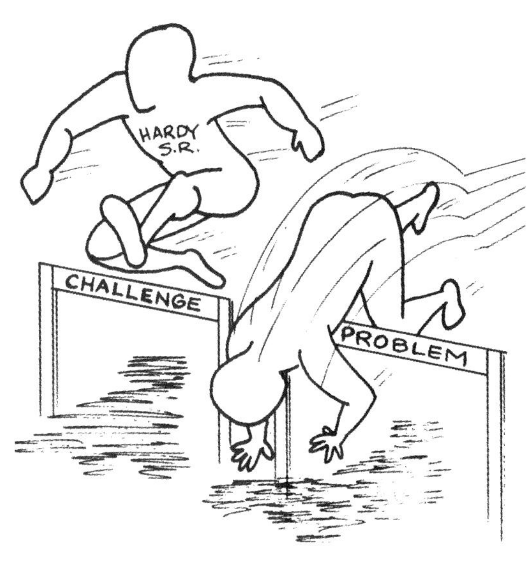

FIGURE 5.9. You can choose to stumble over problems or conquer challenges.

Unnecessary stress in the workplace can come from fearing your job security, having an ill-defined job description, not understanding the function and use of your office equipment (especially computer keyboards and terminals), or not knowing how to effectively deal with customers or clients. Take the time to ask and learn how to perform your job and understand what is expected of you. Reducing or eliminating unknowns, or gray areas in your job description and performance, will significantly reduce your job stress.

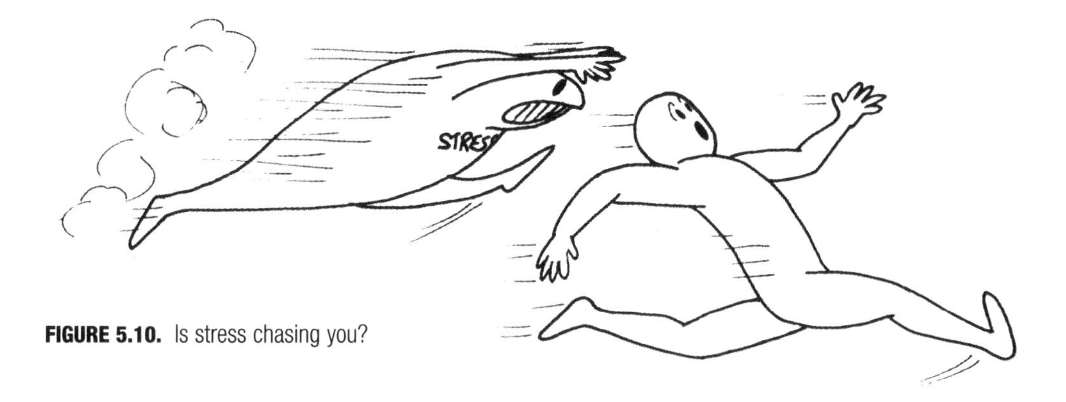

FIGURE 5.10. Is stress chasing you?

Unfinished business on your desk or in your home life can also be a major contributor to the stress that affects you. You may subconsciously think and worry about unfinished business, and this may keep you from releasing stress and its effects when necessary (see Figure 5.10). Complete those projects that you set out to do, or make decisions to put them behind you as possible and practical. Completing your office work can be as mentally exhilarating as finishing a foot race, if you see it that way.

As you can see, stress management is essential to your health as well as to your job performance and satisfaction. It is impossible to explain every aspect of stress in this book. You have a basic understanding, but you may need and want more. There are many good books on the subject, and I encourage you to read and discover more.

You can do a great deal to prevent uncontrolled stress reactions that could otherwise make you ill with headaches, backaches, insomnia, depression, high blood pressure, ulcers, heart disease, and so on. Take the steps necessary to turn this potential enemy into a friend. If you need to, seek professional guidance.

There is no doubt that our lives are and will continue to rapidly change in this day and time. Your ability to survive and succeed is directly related to your ability to see, understand, and adapt to these changes and take care of your body along the way.

6

Exercise

Our ancestors got plenty of exercise just as a matter of survival. They did most of their work by hand and placed great physical demands on their bodies, day after day (see Figure 6.1). Their lives were rigorous, and they had to have strong, hardy bodies to survive. Their exercise requirements were fulfilled by their work.

The "industrial revolution" came, and we began to use machines to make us more productive. Muscle power was no longer the key to survival. The concept of assembly lines came with this era, as we found that it was more efficient to have a worker assemble a small part of a product and perform this assembly many times. Workers learned to perform a task quickly, and companies found that they could make more products and profits this way. This is when a major problem developed. The workers were often using only a small portion of their bodies to do their work. Not only did this strain those parts that were used over and over, but the whole body was not getting the physical exercise it needed.

Now we are on top of the wave of the "information revolution." Modern advancements in communications, computers, and other sophisticated technology have helped create a greater need for the production and delivery of services. Many jobs are available in goods-producing industries, but a greater number of jobs are developing in the office arena. The special requirements of office work and other sedentary occupations usually involve even less movement and physical exertion than work in an industrial plant.

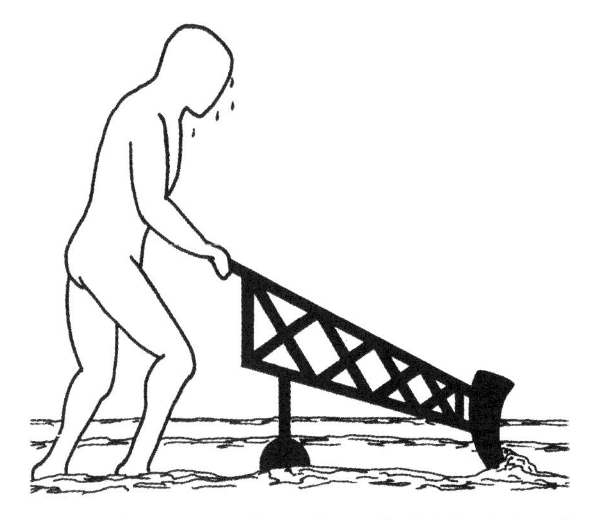

FIGURE 6.1. Our ancestors vigorously exercised during their work.

A typical office worker must sit for a large portion of the workday with a limited ability to move (see Figure 6.2). Sitting, with its special problems, combined with the tense, restrictive effects of stress and doing visually intensive work can inhibit essential, basic physical needs. Bodies were meant to move, and they react badly to this seemingly "easier" lifestyle. Bodies may tend to become fat and soft or overly stressed and tense with unhealthy consequences.

Fortunately, another revolution is paralleling the information revolution. The "fitness" or "wellness" revolution is also upon us, and it has been sorely needed (no pun intended). We are beginning to understand that the ultimate responsibility of our health is in our own hands. We make the decisions to do or not to do the things that keep us vibrant, healthy, and preserve or maintain our health. In the past, we may not have known that we could influence our health and our lives to the extent that we actually can. We now realize that we can choose to either participate and reap the benefits, or just watch and suffer the consequences. The fitness revolution's time has come, and both participants and health scientists agree that regular exercise can produce definite benefits. Many regular exercisers report improved health, feelings of less stress, and greater job satisfaction as a result of their efforts.

Physical exercise is available in many forms and serves many purposes. We will outline how to begin an exercise program, advising you on exercises to do before your workday, during your workday, and during your leisure time. We will also touch on some of the common trouble spots for people who sit most of the time and give you some suggestions.

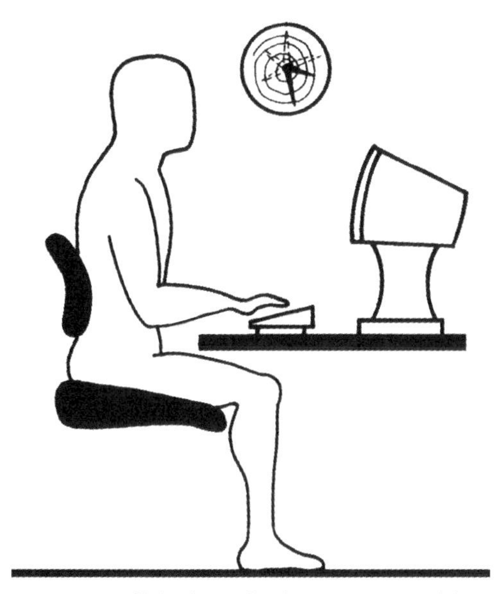

FIGURE 6.2. Sitting hour after hour causes special problems due to limited movement.

If you have a back or joint condition, heart or lung disease, high blood pressure, or have had an injury or surgery, especially if it affects your joints, muscles, ligaments, or vital organs or if you are or have been sedentary or out of shape, it is recommended that you seek qualified professional guidance before starting this or any exercise program.

First of all, let's refresh your memory a little. The underlying framework of your body is the skeleton. The individual bones meet each other to form joints, which are held together by ligaments. Muscles, through contraction and relaxation, move the bones at the joints. The joints are lubricated for smooth and efficient movement, and most joints have a layer of cartilage to keep the bones from rubbing against each other. The spinal vertebrae have a special cushion and shock-absorbing disc between each of them.

Each joint is capable of a particular "range of motion." The combination of all the ranges of motion in the joints of a certain part of your body account for the total range of motion of that particular region. For example, your neck and head are capable of forward, backward, and side bending, as well as rotation by the combination of all of the vertebrae in the neck moving at the joints.

You need to make sure that the joints are moved through their ranges of motion in the proper manner to keep your body flexible. If your joints do not adequately move through their motions, the fluid lubrication cannot be replenished, and the ligaments will slowly tighten and you will begin to lose movement in that joint. The spinal discs need the benefit of regular movement of the vertebrae to replenish and exchange fluids. The combination of lack of regular movement of the vertebrae and the extra pressures produced from long-term sitting, especially with poor chair support or bad postures, can create fixation and misalignment within the joints, all of which can lead to degeneration. Fixation, misalignment, and degeneration produce nerve irritation, and its effects and complications include pain, muscle spasm, fatigue, and organ malfunction.

Requirements of Exercise

The exercise techniques that you choose to use should fulfill several basic body needs. The first is flexibility. Your exercise should move your joints through their normal motions safely and adequately. This concept holds true for general stretching before, during, and after work, as well as warming up and cooling down from more vigorous activities such as aerobic dancing. Next is strength development. Your exercise should stretch, challenge, and strengthen your muscles. You use many muscles in your daily activities, but some are used more than others. All of your muscles need to be regularly used, whether in your work or exercise activities.

Your exercise should condition your body because you sit a great deal of the time at work and probably do not move about vigorously. You need to choose among the exercises that help strengthen the heart, diaphragm, and lungs. Aerobic dancing, bicycling, jogging, swimming, racquetball, tennis, squash, brisk walking, and many other vigorous activities, when done properly, can boost and sustain your heartbeat rate, make you breathe deeply, and cause you to perspire. They help your body utilize oxygen more fully, improve blood cholesterol balance, lower blood pressure, aid in weight control, and help relieve stress and depression.

Finally, your exercise should promote balance and alignment. The exercise programs you use should counteract the effects of long-term sitting and promote equal use of both sides of your body. It should counteract the tension you may feel in your shoulders, arms, neck, back, or legs. Remember, one of the major ways to counteract the detrimental effects of a stressful job is to physically vent the energy and tension that builds up within your body through exercise.

This does not mean you should adopt the "weekend warrior" philosophy and go out to play a vigorous, competitive, three-hour game of tennis on a Saturday afternoon and feel you have exercised enough for the week (see Figure 6.3). This occasional outburst of physical energy on an unconditioned body can actually be harmful and can contribute to physical symptoms you may be experiencing during your office work. Effective exercise should be regular, consistent, and enjoyable.

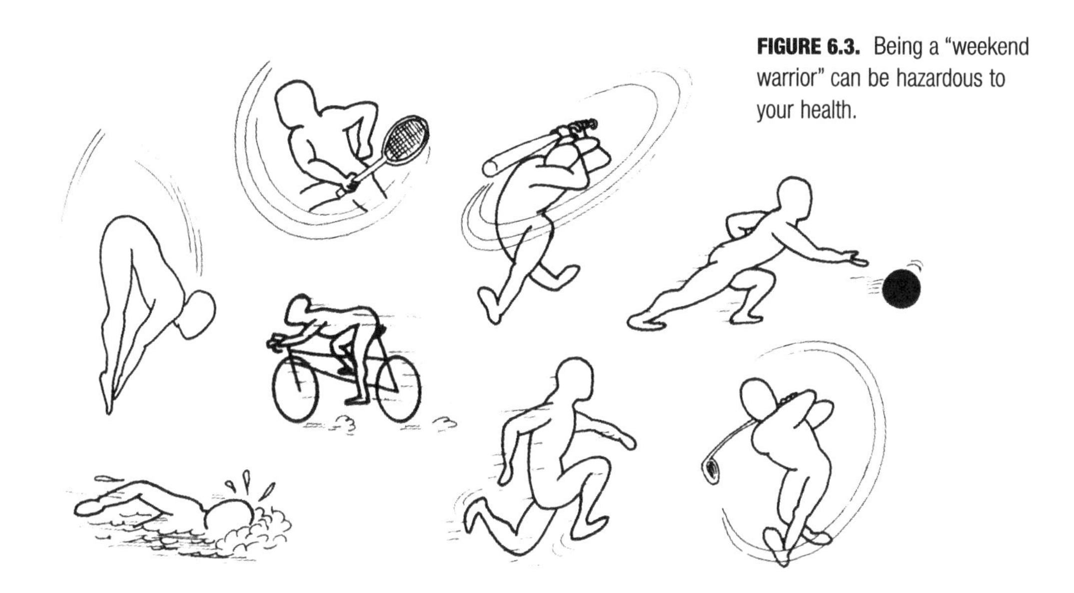

FIGURE 6.3. Being a "weekend warrior" can be hazardous to your health.

Now you are ready to start a program of various exercise activities at work and during your off-work hours. You don't want to go overboard with so many hours of daily exercise that it would sacrifice your home life, but you do want to effectively and efficiently exercise enough to keep your body fit and healthy, because you know how important it is to you and your job performance. The first step is making the commitment to yourself to do the things your body needs.

You now know that your exercise should promote flexibility, strength, conditioning, balance, and alignment. It is important for you to know where and how your body fits into each of these categories as you organize your exercise activities and routines.

Personal Body Inventory

Yes, it's time to look at yourself and take a personal body inventory. Discover your body's present condition, and you will see what areas you need to concentrate on and be able to get started safely. You may need or want professional assistance. Don't risk injuring yourself at this point. Start your personal body inventory by discovering your flexibility or range of motion. Stand in front of a full-length mirror and begin with head and neck movements. Look at the figures on pages 86–88 to see what is considered to be the "normal motions."

Rotate your head slowly to the right and take note where your head stops. Then turn your head to the left, noting where it stops (see Figure 6.4). Pay particular attention to see if one movement is restricted more than the opposite motion. Your goal is to have normal, symmetrical movement. If one movement is much more restricted than the other, carefully review your work and home habits to see if frequent one-sided activities could be a source of the problem. Change your workstation to reduce excessive one-sided movements and postures, and concentrate on stretching the restricted movements to achieve symmetrical motion. If misalignment or fixation has already occurred in the joints, you may need professional assistance to realign or free the fixation so you can safely and beneficially proceed with your exercises.

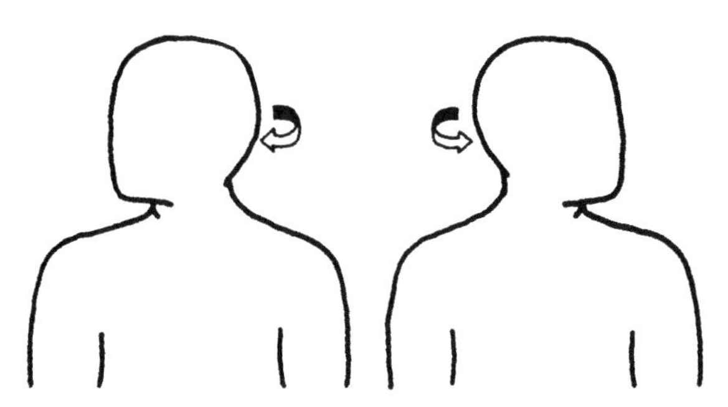

FIGURE 6.4. Head rotation is usually eighty degrees to the left and to the right.

Tilt your head to the right, making sure you keep your nose straight ahead. Note this motion as well as the movement of your head and neck tilting to the left (see Figure 6.5). Look for uneven motion either way. Bend your head forward toward your chest, comparing your motion with the normal movement (see Figure 6.6). Repeat the process as you tilt your head slowly backward. If any of these movements create pain or make you lightheaded or dizzy, you should seek professional assistance.

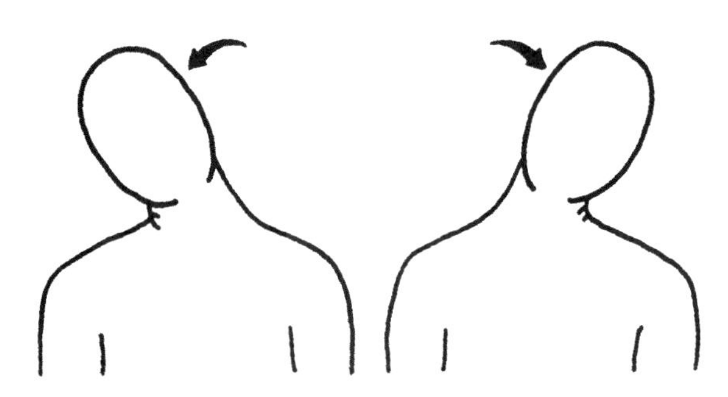

FIGURE 6.5. Head side tilting is normally forty-five degrees to the left and to the right.

Look for painful and/or restricted motion during all movements of your neck, back, shoulders, arms, hands, legs, and feet. Pain is usually an indication of trouble and should be professionally evaluated before getting involved in an exercise program.

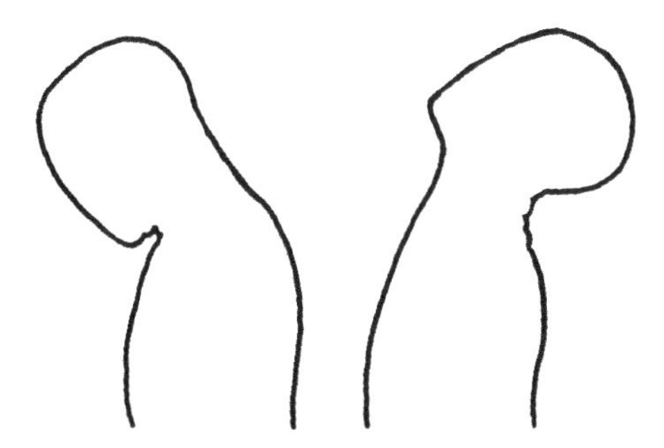

FIGURE 6.6. Normally a person can tilt their head far enough forward to touch their chin to their chest and backward far enough to look at the ceiling directly above them.

Stay in front of the mirror and compare your body motion with the "normal" movements illustrated in Figures 6.7, 6.8, and 6.9. It's important to mention that some people are not physically able to move their bodies through the "normal" range of motion, even after a great deal of work. Some of this restriction could be due to unique joint formations or a previous injury or surgery, so don't strain yourself or feel like a failure if you can't achieve what is considered "normal motion." You are already improving yourself through your efforts. If you run into problems or have questions, ask a doctor who specializes in the evaluation and treatment of these type of disorders.

You should also check your shoulder, arm, wrist, finger, leg, knee, ankle, and foot motions. Illustrations of these motions are not included in this book, but you should check for unrestricted, painless, symmetrical motion in these joints. Remember, obvious restriction may mean the joints have not been exercised for a long time, or may be traced back to work or home habits, or a previous injury or surgery. Be careful of pain when stretching or exercising.

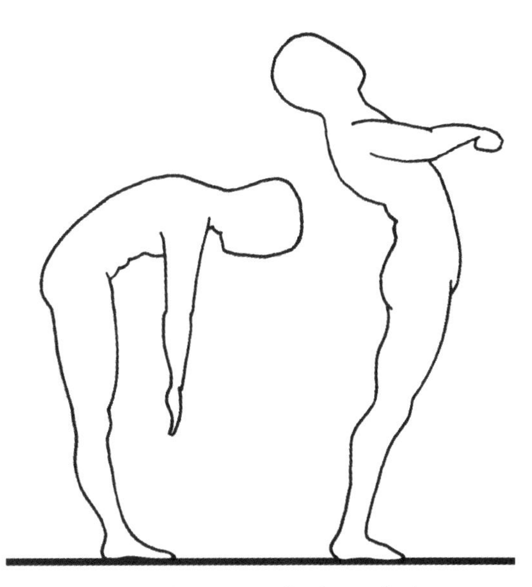

FIGURE 6.7. Forward bending is usually about ninety degrees and backward bending is usually about thirty degrees.

A fit body is flexible but is also strong and well conditioned. Muscles need to be challenged or worked to remain strong and healthy. The characteristics of prolonged sitting with limited movement in office or sedentary work pose a special challenge. The postural muscles involved in sitting get

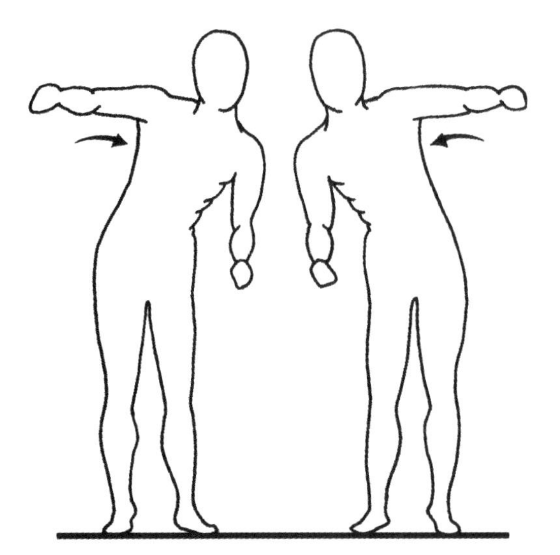

FIGURE 6.8. Side bending is normally about thirty degrees in each direction.

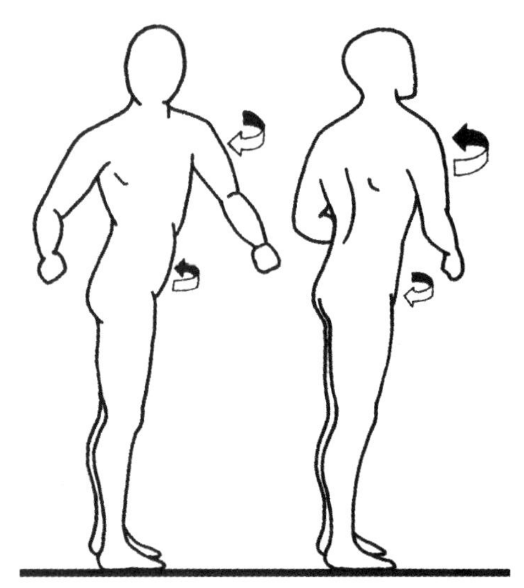

FIGURE 6.9. Trunk rotation is normally thirty degrees or greater in each direction.

adequate challenge during the day. However, if you sit improperly at your workstation, or don't use your chair for maximum support, these muscles will become overworked and strained. Meanwhile, other muscles are not working or being challenged. If you don't take measures to work these muscles, weakness and imbalance can occur.

Adequate and proper stretching is a very important part of exercise and fitness. An excellent book to read is *Stretching* by Bob Anderson.

Special Hazards of Sitting

Jan Beckwith, creator and president of Body Flex, Inc., in Lincoln, Nebraska, has been a remarkable innovator in the application of aerobic exercise. She has developed a thirty-minute workout involving warm-up, aerobic, and cool-down exercise. Many office workers utilize her program before work, during lunch, or after work to stretch, condition, and strengthen their bodies, as well as to vent and counteract the stresses and strains they encounter in their work. They find the program effective and enjoyable. Mrs. Beckwith has made several observations about the general physical problems sedentary workers experience. People who sit a great deal tend to develop weak abdominal, buttock, and front and inner thigh muscles (see Figure 6.10). Their neck, shoulder, and back

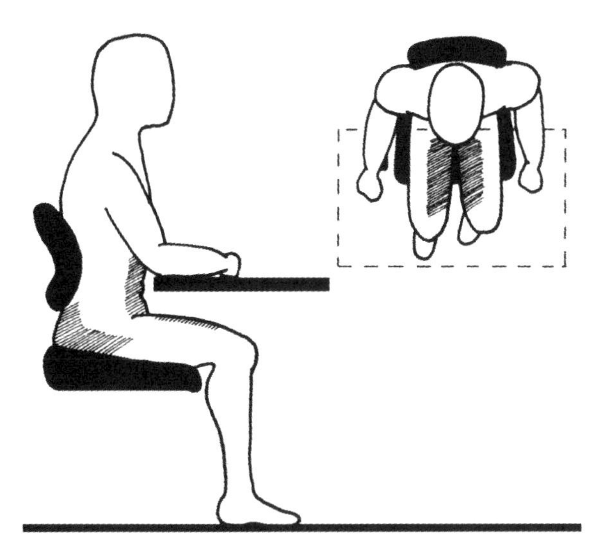

FIGURE 6.10. Abdominal, buttock, and front and inner thigh muscles are frequent trouble spots for people who sit.

muscles tend to be tense, and their spinal movements are usually restricted.

When you sit, your thighs come up toward your body and because your body is erect, the abdominal muscles relax. They relax even more if you lean over your desk to do your work. The foot, lower leg, and back thigh muscles can be stretched and exercised while sitting, but the front and inner thigh muscles cannot be adequately stretched. As you sit, your buttock muscles bear the weight of your upper body and they are difficult to stretch while sitting. You can see how problems can develop in these critical areas. You must make sure these major muscle groups get the stretching, strengthening, and conditioning they need through your exercise programs, or major structural imbalances will occur in your body, and, over time, you will suffer the consequences.

Your body functions as a whole, and if you use only certain parts, they may become overly strained, while the lesser used parts become weak. Many problems can develop this way. I mentioned in the introduction that knowledge is power, and you now are gaining the knowledge to understand the physical problems that can arise from sitting and performing your work. You can use this knowledge, and with proper work habits, postures, stress management, and exercise, you can neutralize or reverse the negative effects of sitting on the job.

Let's learn how you can use stretching and exercising to your advantage. We will use the example of properly playing a game of tennis. First, you have selected good, supportive shoes to wear, and you are wearing comfortable, nonrestrictive clothing. You have a tennis racquet that is sized and strung to accommodate your type of play, and the handle was chosen to fit your hand and grip. You have probably taken lessons to learn how to make smooth and easy, but powerful and accurate, swings in a way that won't strain or injure you. Before the match, you warm up by stretching all of your leg, back, neck, shoulder, arm, and hand muscles and joints. You also make several practice serves and swings so you will have the proper timing.

Now you're ready to play. You concentrate and focus your attention on the tennis ball, your opponent, his or her style of play, and your own game plan. When the ball comes into your court, your body tenses a bit as you move to the ball to make your shot. Between points, you relax for a moment and stretch some of your muscles as you walk back to position. Between games, you spend a little more time to take a few deep breaths and stretch while you are thinking about your strategy. Between sets, you relax and stretch a little more as you towel off. Then you take a few more deep breaths, and mentally and physically prepare for the next set. You have learned how to stretch and relax while still concentrating on your game.

When the match is over, you walk to the net and thank your opponent for a good game. If you are wise, you will then do a series of cool-down stretches to keep your joints limber and let your muscles slowly unwind from the exercise and challenge you have given them. You take a warm, relaxing shower, get dressed, and leave. The game should have been enjoyable whether you won or lost the match. You win by giving your body vital physical exercise.

Throughout this sporting activity, though it was strenuous and demanding, you took many breaks of varying lengths to refresh your body. At the same time, you were still able to concentrate on the match. Can you imagine how hard it would be for you to stay tight and tense during the entire match? You would wear down quickly, and it probably wouldn't be much fun. Can you see how the same thing can happen to you at work? If you are tight and tense during the entire day and don't take the time to stretch, relax, and refresh your mind and body, you will wear down. Your productivity, accuracy, and consistency will suffer, and you won't get the satisfaction that you should from performing your job well. You are also more likely to suffer from some of the physical symptoms that were discussed earlier in this book. There are many things you can do to control your condition.

Exercising Your Way Through the Workday

Let's take the concepts we discussed in the tennis match and transfer them to your office work. After all, your work can be considered a sport. Yes, a sport can be broadly defined as any physical activity engaged in for pleasure and personal benefit. Your work does require physical movements, as well as the physical effort of sitting. You should obtain pleasure from overcoming the challenges and stress of your tasks, as well as a sense of accomplishment from successfully performing your job and helping in the operation of a business. Personal benefit also comes from getting paid for your efforts so you can provide for yourself and your family.

Now that we have oriented our thoughts to view work as a sport, let's stretch, relax, and exercise ourselves through one day's events. You may be able to develop a rhythm in your work activities and stretch and exercise during breaks as described below. The day starts when you get out of bed. You take a few moments to slowly stretch your neck, back, arms, and legs before you shower, eat breakfast, or dress for work. If you are a morning person and an early riser, you may choose to do some type of vigorous exercise, such as jogging, swimming, or aerobics after your morning stretches.

On your way to work, you mentally prepare yourself for the day's tasks. You think about what needs to be done and how you are going to do it efficiently. You walk to your workstation, standing erect and feeling good, and look around to see if the equipment, materials, work surface, and chair are arranged and adjusted to fit your body to the task. If they are not, you make the necessary changes and adjustments. You have probably been well trained in the use of your particular office equipment, so you can efficiently perform your tasks with less stress. You sit down and begin your work activities.

There are usually many times throughout the day when you can counteract some of the tension and strain that builds up while you work. This can be done in much the same way as our tennis player who took breaks of varying degrees during the match. We will call them micro breaks, mini breaks, macro breaks, and lunch breaks. Let's look at each one of these breaks and see how you can effectively use them.

Micro Breaks

Micro breaks are very important and can be frequently used to effectively counteract tension buildup and fatigue in the muscles and eyes. The break may only be momentary or last up to a minute. If you have a visually demanding task, you can use a few quick and easy exercises several times an hour to reduce strain. You can change your focus by looking at an object that is more than twenty feet away. Look out the window or at a picture on a relatively distant wall. If you sit at a workstation surrounded by room dividers, look up at the ceiling or lean back and look outside the room dividers, but make sure you don't excessively crane your neck.

Your eyes may benefit from taking a break from the lights in the room or from your computer screen. Take a moment to lightly place the palms of your hands over your eyes while they are closed (see Figure 6.11). Hold this position for thirty to sixty seconds. Avoid pressing your palms into your eyeballs. If you find that you are always looking in one direction while performing your tasks, take a moment to look in the other direction. This gives you a chance to exercise eye and neck muscles that are used less frequently.

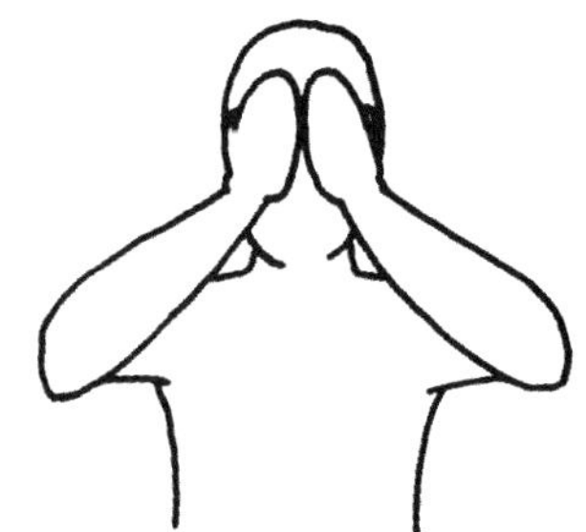

FIGURE 6.11. Take frequent vision breaks.

If you do a considerable amount of work with your hands on a keyboard, typewriter, calculator, or telephone, you may need to frequently exercise and stretch your fingers, hands, wrists, and forearms. Shrug your shoulders up toward your ears or roll your shoulders backward and forward in circular motions (see Figure 6.12). Turn your head slowly to one side, then to the other, or tilt your head slowly to one shoulder then to the other.

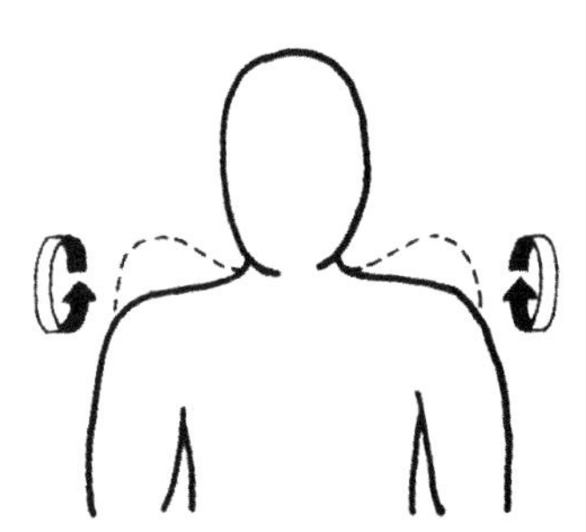

FIGURE 6.12. Shrugging your shoulders in circular motions will help the muscles relax.

If you are performing a stressful task, you may need to take a moment to take a deep breath or two. Be sure to slowly breathe in through your nose (unless you have a cold) and slowly out through your mouth. This breathing exercise gives your body more oxygen and helps relax the rib cage and upper body.

If you sit for long periods of time, take a moment to check and adjust your posture or push back into your chair's back support to stretch. You can also stretch your leg muscles by straightening your legs and moving your ankles and feet (see Figure 6.13). You should have enough room under the work surface to move your legs about. Stray or dangling cords and wires need to

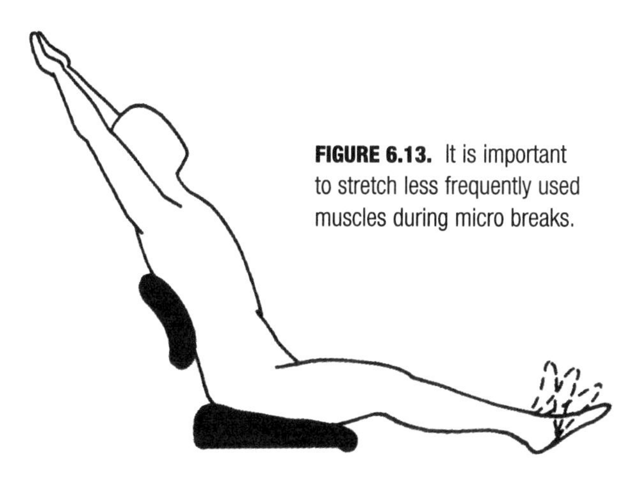

FIGURE 6.13. It is important to stretch less frequently used muscles during micro breaks.

be attached to the wall or moved out of the way. Personal items, such as purses, books, and coats under the work surface, should not hinder leg movement.

You won't be able to do all of these exercises during each micro break. Just use the ones that pertain to the type of work you do. You can alternate them, or use some and not others, according to what your body needs and responds to best. Don't consume your workday with breaks, or excessively interrupt the flow of your work. You want to use breaks to refresh your body and improve your comfort and productivity.

Mini Breaks

Mini breaks should occur less frequently, but will give you more time to combine a couple of different exercises or do more repetitions of the deep breathing, body stretches, or eye exercises. Mini breaks can be used during a natural lull in your work activities. You have a little more time during a mini break, so you may want to push your chair away from the work surface and bend over to stretch your back muscles (see Figure 6.14), or sit and pull one knee toward your chest and hold it for five seconds and do the same with the other leg (see Figure 6.15). To be effective, this should be repeated four to six times.

An exercise known as the "cat stretch" may be appropriate here or during macro breaks (see Figure 6.16). Stand up at your workstation and place your hands on your work surface at about shoulder width. Your feet should also be about shoulder width from each other. Slowly arch your back like a cat, dropping your head toward your chest while tucking your pelvis inward. Hold this position for a couple of seconds. Then bow your lower back downward while pushing your buttocks backward and raising your head toward the ceiling. Hold this position for a couple of seconds. To be effective, this exercise should be repeated five to ten times. This exercise should not be painful.

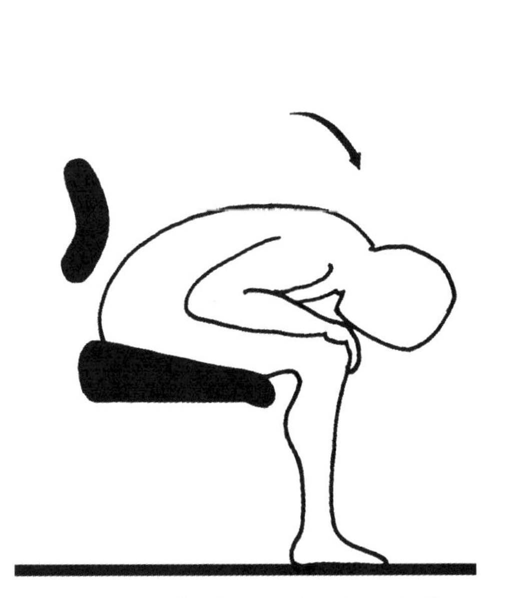

FIGURE 6.14. Bend over to stretch your back muscles.

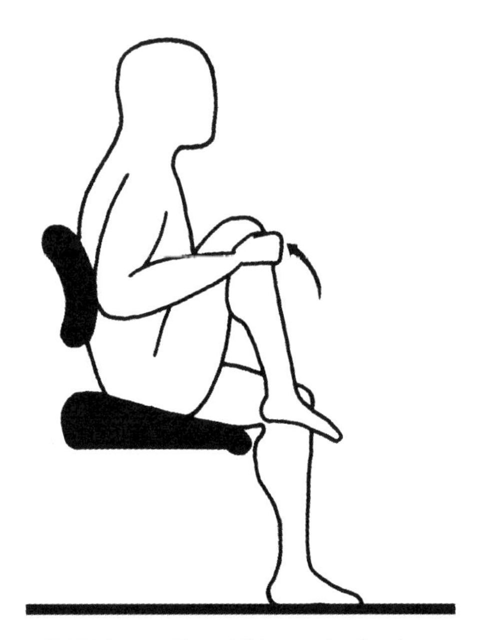

FIGURE 6.15. Repeat this exercise four to six times for each leg.

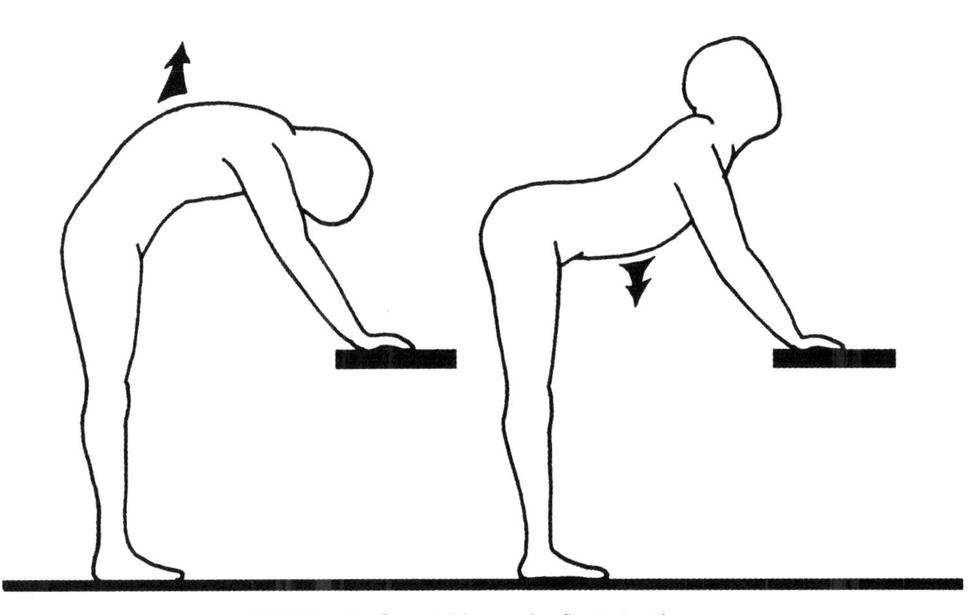

FIGURE 6.16. Repeat this exercise five to ten times.

Macro Breaks

Macro breaks are the well-known scheduled coffee breaks. You may have ten to fifteen minutes, and you may have the chance to get out of your chair and stretch or socialize with your coworkers. You may be able to perform the "cat stretch" exercise at this time. This may be an ideal time to divert your concentration and give your mind a break from your tasks. It's also a good time to use some of the stress-reduction techniques discussed in Chapter 5. You can use positive imagery or take a stress and strain inventory of your body and do the appropriate exercises to counteract their effects.

Lunch Breaks

Lunch breaks last from thirty to sixty minutes and you may use this time to eat, do some shopping, run errands, or exercise. Many large companies provide exercise facilities for their employees. If your firm does, take advantage of this provision over lunch or before or after work. You may be able to go swimming, jogging, cycling, aerobic dancing, or play racquetball at the local YMCA or YWCA.

Remember that the vigorous exercise activities you choose should follow the guidelines discussed earlier in this chapter. If you sit at your workstation for most of the day, you should do something other than sit for your entire lunch break. If you are too tired to do anything but sit, it is a strong indication that something is wrong.

Now you have an idea how to use your breaks throughout the day to reduce stress and strain, to refresh your body and mind, and to make yourself more comfortable and productive in your work. The next step is making the commitment to use these breaks effectively, and taking action to do it consistently. It's simply a matter of forming the right habits.

After your workday, you can do many things that you can't do in the office to help your body unwind and reduce the effects of stress and strain. You can practice more involved stress-reduction techniques, such as progressive relaxation. You should also do an enjoyable, vigorous exercise activity that has an aerobic effect at least three to four times each week. If you are out of shape or have special circumstances, check with your doctor before you start. You may need to gradually work up to this level. You may be more likely to regularly and consistently exercise if you engage in organized workouts or sports with other people.

Special Exercises

There are also a few special exercises you should use to help counteract the physical effects of sitting. They involve the abdominal, buttock, and front and inner thigh muscles, and an area in the back just several inches below the shoulder blades. Study the figures and explanations so you can perform these exercises safely and effectively. Seek professional assistance if you have questions or special circumstances. Be sure to perform these exercises on a carpeted or padded floor.

The abdominal muscles are among the first muscles to become weak from sitting for long periods of time. The reverse sit-up (see Figure 6.17) is a safe and effective way to exercise and begin to strengthen these muscles. Lie on your back with your arms at your sides and palms downward. Bend your knees and place your feet firmly on the floor. Slowly raise your bent legs upward past your breast line or above your face. Slowly return your legs and feet to the starting position. Repeat this exercise five to ten times.

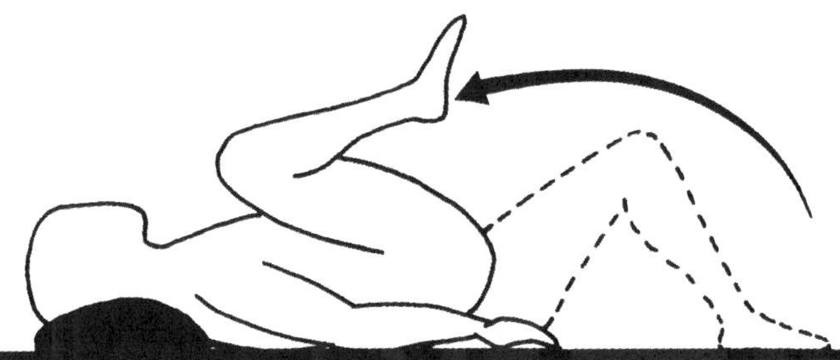

FIGURE 6.17. Repeat this exercise five to ten times.

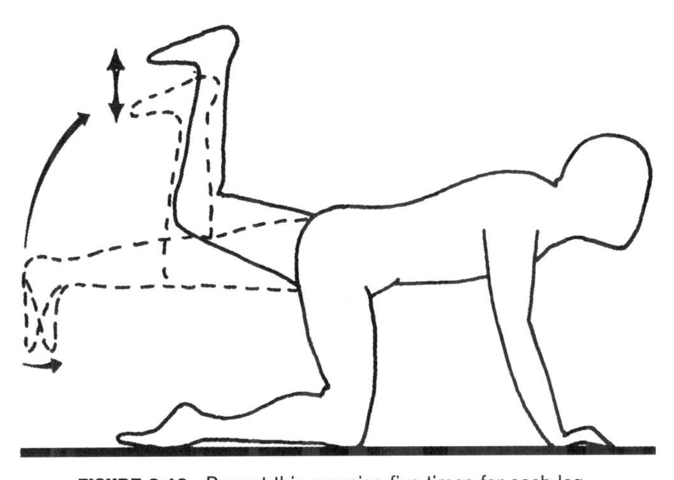

FIGURE 6.18. Repeat this exercise five times for each leg.

To help stretch and

exercise the buttock muscles that you sit on all day, try the following exercise (see Figure 6.18). Get down on your hands and knees and spread them apart at about shoulder width. Extend your left leg backward and lift it upward while keeping your back straight. Flex your foot toward your shin and bend your knee. Push your heel upward, toward the ceiling, using slow short lifts always returning to hip level. Repeat this exercise five times if it does not become uncomfortable. Repeat the entire procedure on the right side. You can do more than five repetitions with each leg if it is comfortable and not too tiring.

The thigh muscles also need help if you sit for long periods of time. Lie on your back with your upper body supported by your elbows (see Figure 6.19). Keep your lower back pressed toward the floor. Cross your ankles and slowly raise your legs toward the ceiling while keeping your lower back and hips pressed to the floor. When your legs are vertical, slowly spread your ankles three to four feet apart without arching your back or dropping your hips. Bring your legs together and cross your ankles the opposite way. Do not bend your knees. Repeat this exercise five to ten times if comfortable.

The front thigh muscles also need to be regularly stretched. Stand with your right shoulder a couple of inches away from a wall and place your right hand on the wall or a stationary chair (see Figure 6.20). Pull your left ankle backward and grab it with your left hand. Roll your shoulders forward so that your lower back is straight. Slowly bend forward, using the support of the chair or wall, while pulling your left ankle upward. You will begin to feel a stretching sensation in your left thigh. Hold at a comfortable stretching position for five seconds. Return to the upright position and repeat this procedure five times. Do the same on the opposite side.

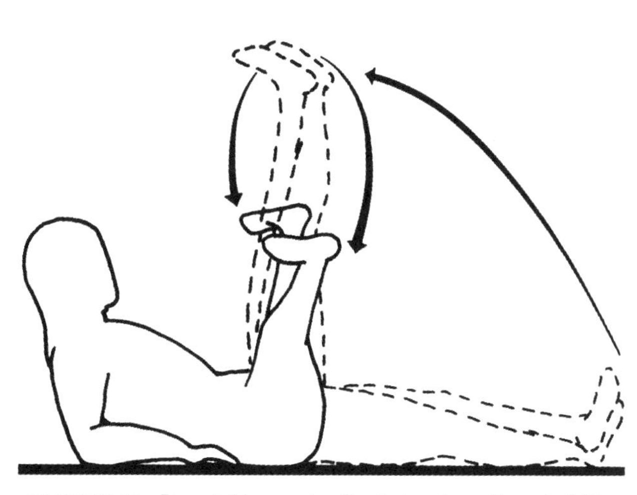

FIGURE 6.19. Repeat this exercise five to ten times if comfortable.

The next exercise helps stretch and relax that part of your back that bears a great deal of stress and strain when you lean forward in your chair and do not have the backrest to support you. Roll an ordinary bath towel so that it is about two inches in diameter. Sit on the floor with your legs extended. Place the towel at the spot in your spine just above the forward curve of your lower back and several inches below your shoulder blades. Lie down on your back with the towel in this position and relax for two to three minutes (see Figure 6.21). This helps stretch and relax the part of your back that bears a great deal of stress when you lean forward in your chair and do not have the backrest to support you.

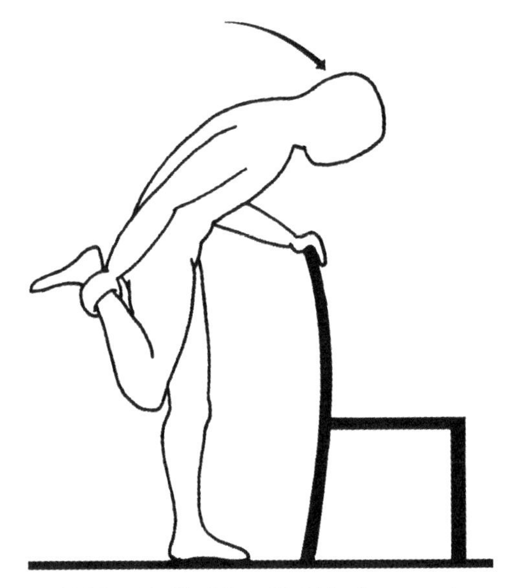

FIGURE 6.20. Stretch and hold for five seconds. Alternate legs five times each.

We have concentrated on exercising your body both during work and outside of work, but one final point is important to mention. The mind and body work so closely together that it is essential that you exercise your mind as well as your body. I close this chapter with a quote from Dr. Howard H. Jan from his 1986 *Success Journal*:

> Your mind, like your muscles, can either be agile or allowed to grow flabby through lack of use. Atrophy of the mind happens when you always do the same old things in the same old way, without any challenges to your mind. To exercise your mind, do something new, something different, take a walk through the woods, go to a concert, to a museum, see a thought-provoking movie, read a controversial book. Take a different route to work, eat exotic meals. Take up a new hobby or sport.

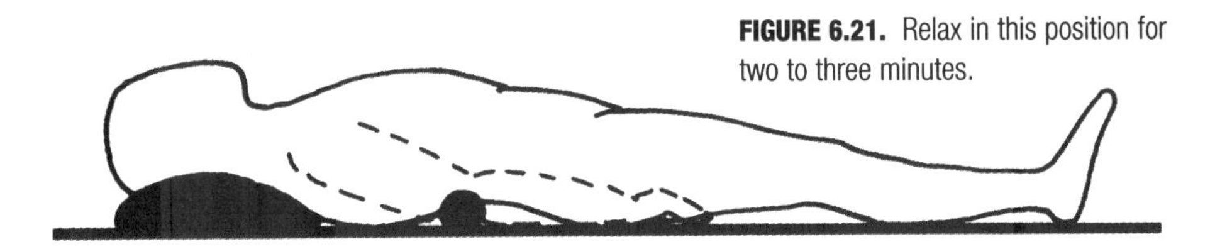

FIGURE 6.21. Relax in this position for two to three minutes.

7

Sleep

During an average week, you may be spending about as much time sleeping as you do working, so it is important to describe some of the characteristics of sleep and what positions are best for your body. During periods of rest and sleep, your body tries to counteract the effects of the stress and strains of your day. It charges your battery and rejuvenates you to help you face life's coming events with enthusiasm and positive expectations. If you wake up tired and tense, it is difficult to start the day with a positive attitude.

First, let's review some facts about sleep. One of the most important facts is that it's not the quantity of sleep, but the quality of sleep you get each night that counts most. Studies by sleep scientists have shown that people can reduce their normal sleeping time by up to two and one-half hours nightly without suffering ill effects or daytime sleepiness. If you are average, this means you are probably getting enough sleep, but you should make every minute of this time work for the benefit of you and your body.

Sleep should be an enjoyable time (see Figure 7.1). It satisfies our deep instinctive need to feel safe and secure. We usually feel we need more sleep when we are depressed or under a great deal of stress. Sleep disorders, restless

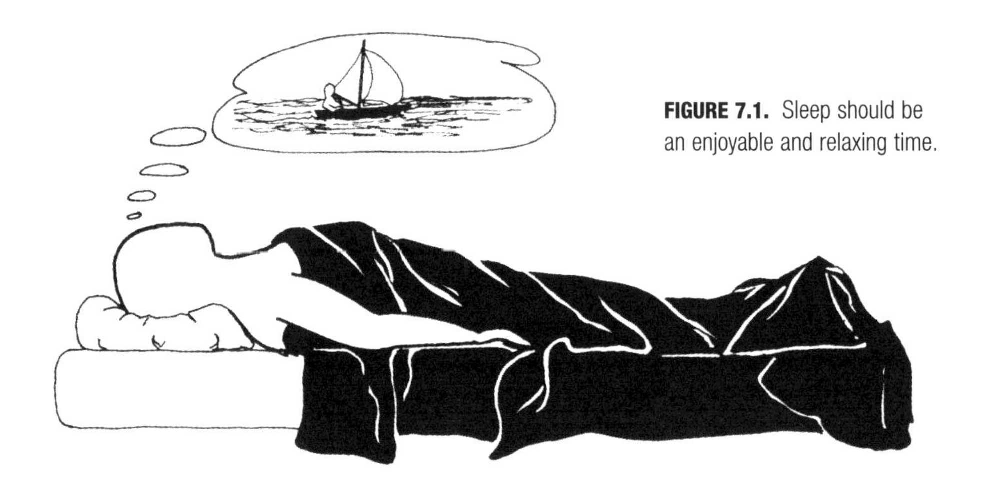

FIGURE 7.1. Sleep should be an enjoyable and relaxing time.

or fitful sleeping habits, or poor sleeping postures can contribute to or aggravate many physical conditions such as fibrositis and degenerative arthritis, spinal misalignment, and muscle and ligament strain. These factors may directly or indirectly contribute to back and neck aches, headaches, and other pains or symptoms you experience while performing your work. So let's consider ways to increase the quality of your sleep and then focus on proper sleeping postures.

The normal sleep cycle lasts about ninety minutes. This includes the several periods of light sleep that gradually lead to very deep sleep and then back again to a light sleep. Most of us have experienced the tired, groggy feeling we get when waking during deep sleep. It's hard to get started, and we feel "off" the entire day. It's important to try to work with our own individual sleep cycles. The following research and clinically proven methods might help you improve the quality of your sleep.

First, schedule your "sleep time" with your own sleep rhythms. A period of drowsiness brought on by a lowering of body temperature to about 97 degrees precedes sleep, whether it is ten minutes or ten hours. If you work with your natural cycle, you will probably get your best quality rest whether it is a full night's sleep or a refreshing nap. If your drowsy period occurs at 2:30 A.M. instead of the nation's customary bedtime of 11:00 P.M., your quality of sleep for four hours may be more beneficial to you than eight hours of tossing and turning.

Contrary to popular desire, it may be better for you to resist the temptation for that Saturday or Sunday morning sleep-in. By getting up at the same time every morning, you reset your body clock and recycle all your sleep and wake cycles. Waking up late one day may throw off your next day's cycles. Early morning drowsiness can be overcome by thinking about a high-interest activity.

Sleep scientists disagree on the value of taking daytime naps. Some believe naps decrease the quantity of nighttime sleep, and they are usually impractical during our workday. There is, however, an impressive number of sixty-hour-a-week executives, as well as historic figures, who attest to the value of daytime dozing or catnaps when drowsy periods hit. Napoleon, Winston Churchill, and Presidents Truman, Johnson, and Kennedy were some of the most famous nappers. It was said of Thomas Edison, who averaged only three hours of sleep a night: "His secret weapon was the catnap. His genius for sleep equaled his genius for invention."

Stay on a regular schedule as much as possible. Eat balanced meals at regular times and make sure your body gets the important nutrients it needs for optimum health. Exercise regularly, but, if you exercise late in the afternoon or in the evening, make it light. Exercising too vigorously late in the evening may be overstimulating. Take care of any physical condition, including headaches, and back and neck pains that interrupt sleep. Stress carried over from the day's activities may cause poor sleep, so you may want to practice relaxing, stress-reduction techniques at bedtime. Mild body stretching may also be relaxing.

Be cautious about using drugs to help you sleep. Sleep-inducing drugs should be used only under careful supervision and in special cases. Using them on your own for long periods may allow residues of the drug in your body to carry over into the daytime and cause dull thinking as well as slow reflexes. If you decide to use these drugs, be careful as they can create a dangerous cycle. You may feel drowsy and tired during the day and reach for that third, fourth, or tenth cup of coffee, tea, or other caffeinated beverage in order to stay awake. Then at night you will be wired from the caffeine and will reach for more sleeping pills. This artificially induced sleep and wakefulness cycle can have devastating effects on your body and your job performance. Don't let this happen to you. Seek professional assistance if necessary.

Alcoholic "nightcaps" can be almost as harmful to your health. Sleep produced by alcohol, a depressant, is of poor quality. There is little deep or dreaming sleep, and frequent awakenings are common, both from withdrawal as the body metabolizes the alcohol and from the need to get up to go the bathroom. The drug nicotine is a central nervous system stimulant, so if you smoke or chew tobacco, stop well before bedtime. Smokers who quit completely often experience dramatic improvements in the quality of their sleep. Skip that middle-of-the-evening cup of caffeinated coffee, tea, or cola, as well. The stimulating effects of the caffeine in these drinks last at least six hours. Chocolate and many common pain relievers also contain caffeine and may affect the quality and quantity of your sleep.

The environment you sleep in is also important. Make it as quiet, dark, and comfortable as possible. You may find it better to sleep in a slightly cool, but not cold, room. A room temperature in the mid-sixties may be best, but make sure that you don't have drafts or fans blowing on your body. Your mattress should be large and firm enough for comfort. Some people prefer waterbeds instead of conventional bedding as their choice of sleep support. This decision should be made by you with the help of a trusted and knowledgeable healthcare professional who has a thorough understanding of your body's mechanics.

Relax before you go to bed. Don't go to bed with your day's problems on your mind. The primary purpose of sleep is to relax your body and prepare you for the next day's activities, so don't carry stress into your sleep; it will only accumulate within you. A good night's sleep will allow you to start fresh each day. Take an hour before bedtime to wind down and do something you enjoy. Try reading in the proper postures (not in bed—see Figure 7.2), watching TV, listening to or playing music, or working on an enjoyable hobby (as long as it doesn't cause you stress or body strain).

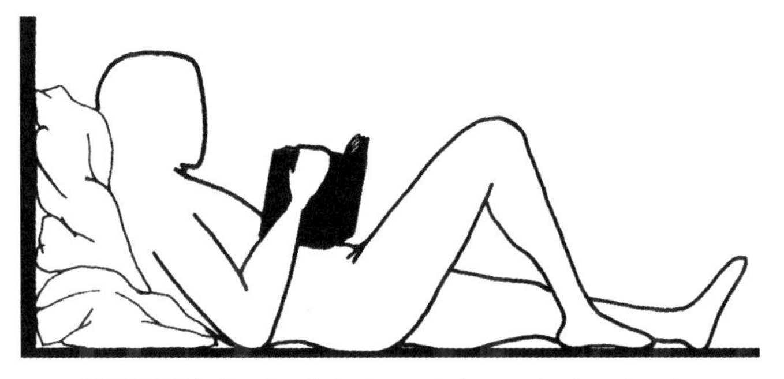

FIGURE 7.2. Reading in bed can strain your back and neck.

If you wish, and your diet can afford it, have a light snack before bedtime. Research shows that people are sleepier after a high-carbohydrate snack than after one containing high protein. Try a glass of milk or other noncaffeine, nonalcoholic drink, a dish of breakfast cereal or a light sandwich. It's best to avoid peanuts, beans, and most raw fruits and vegetables, as they can cause gas. High-fat or deep-fried snacks, such as potato or corn chips, should also be avoided as they can keep your digestive system overactive.

Your inner clock will be reminded of sleep if you follow a regular routine each night before retiring. A ritual such as brushing your teeth, washing your face, setting the alarm, and turning off the lights may help signal your body to sleep. Try to follow your ritual even when you are away from home. Don't go to bed if you aren't sleepy. If you still have problems on your mind, try reading a boring or difficult book until you become sleepy (see Figure 7.3). If your muscles feel as if they are tied up in knots, relax them with the techniques described in Chapter 5.

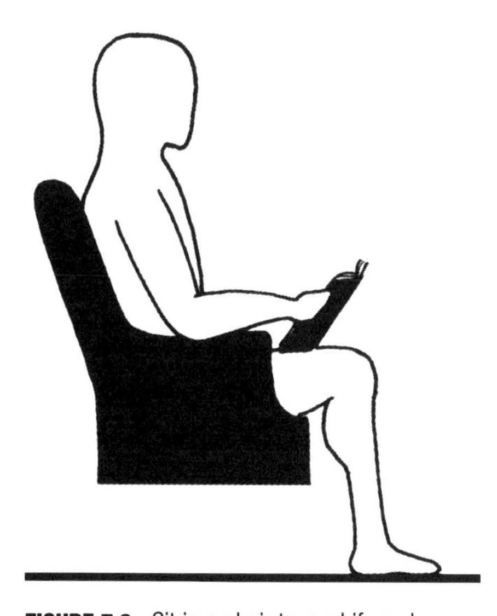

FIGURE 7.3. Sit in a chair to read if you have difficulty falling asleep.

Relax in bed by stretching your body and getting comfortable. Get a feeling of relaxation and warmth. Pleasant imagery can also help. Imagine yourself in a relaxing scene. Let your thoughts float and don't concentrate too much on any one subject, especially about forcing yourself to fall asleep. Think about good and pleasant things that are happening in your life, as long as they do not get you too excited. If you aren't asleep in twenty minutes or so, don't just lie there and worry and fight it. Get out of bed and go into another room. Continue relaxing activities until you are sleepy. Wait for your drowsy period before going to bed again.

Proper Sleeping Postures

Now you know how important the quality of your sleep is and several ways to help you maximize its effects, but it is also important that you understand and use proper sleeping postures (see Figure 7.4). You may toss and turn in your sleep much like you move about while sitting in your chair at work. It's normal to move and shift in your chair, even if your body has proper support and you use good postures. Likewise, it's normal to toss and turn while sleeping (see

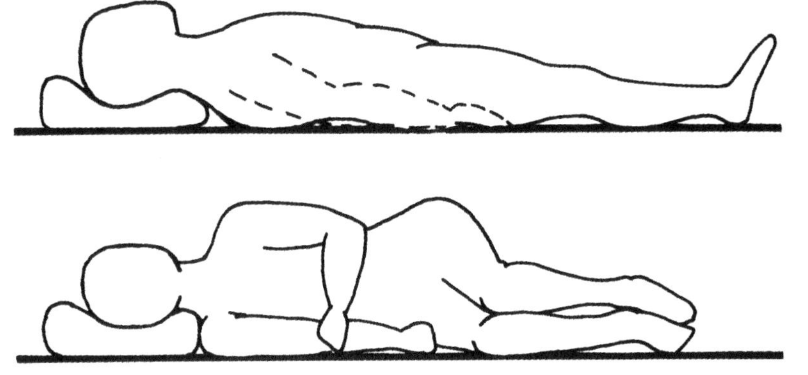

FIGURE 7.4. Proper sleeping positions.

Figure 7.5), but you should have a good, supportive mattress and pillow, and you should use proper sleeping postures.

When you are sitting upright, the forces of gravity are pulling down on the bones and discs of your spine, and your muscles and ligaments are working to support you (see Figure 7.6). During sleep, you are horizontal and gravity is no longer compressing the length of your body (see Figure 7.7). You need relief from the effects of gravity to maintain a healthy body, so the bedding you

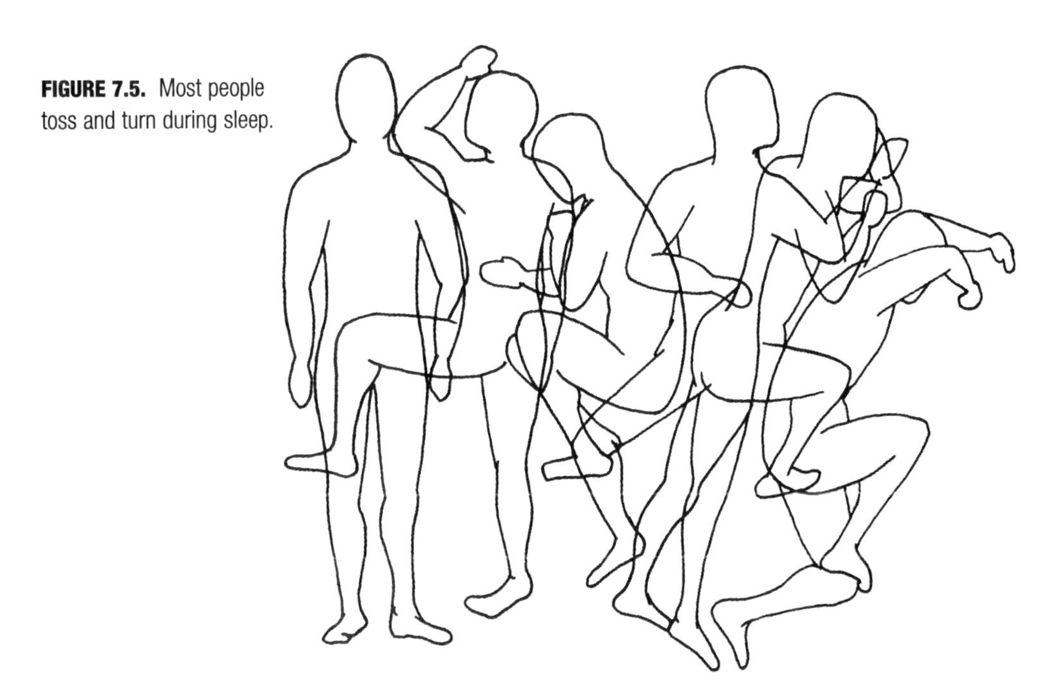

FIGURE 7.5. Most people toss and turn during sleep.

choose must support the weight of your body without sagging, and yet be pliable enough to accommodate the contours of your spine, hips, shoulders, neck, and head. A sagging mattress or inadequately filled waterbed places extra strain on your body when you are supposed to be relaxed and supported. This prevents your body from erasing or reducing the strains and pressures it goes through during the day, and you will end up carrying this strain and pressure into the next day's activities. The cumulative effect of this carryover can aggravate many of the problems you experience during your work and other daily activities.

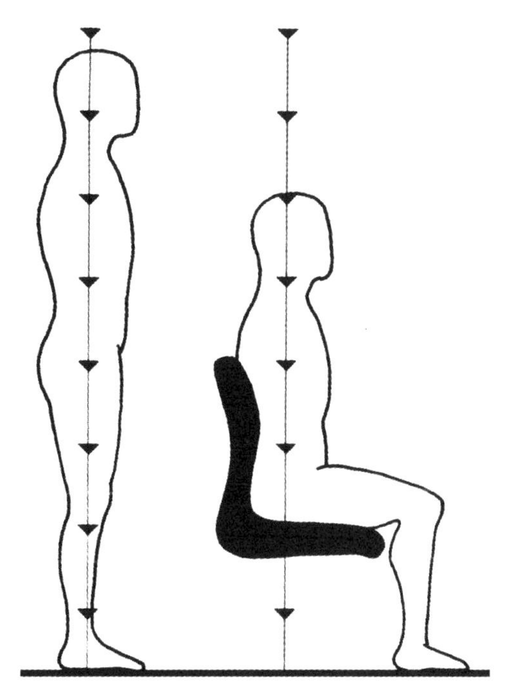

FIGURE 7.6. Gravity is constantly affecting your body while standing and sitting.

In previous chapters, we described the negative effects that too much twisting or turning in one direction can have on your spinal, muscular, and ligament balance, and how it can cause misalignment and nerve irritation. The same thing holds true for sleeping postures. If you sleep on your stomach most of the time, the curve of your lower

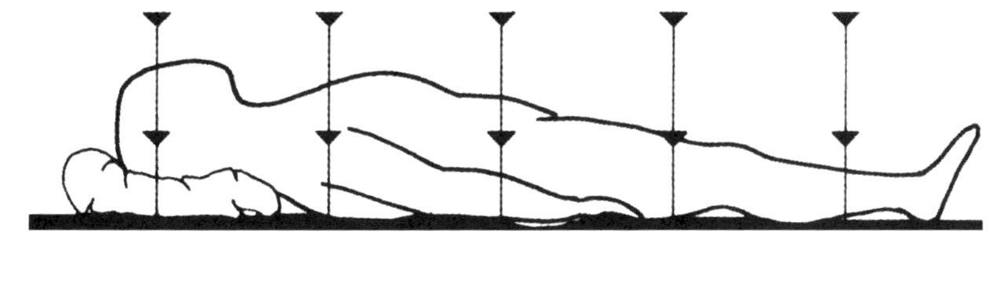

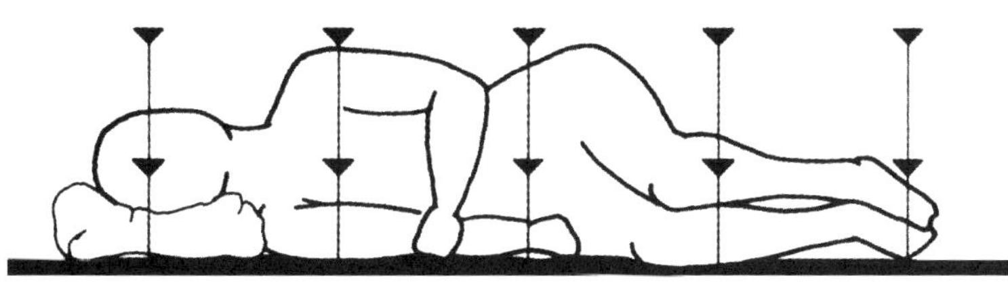

FIGURE 7.7. Proper sleeping postures reduce gravity's effects on your body.

back is strained (see Figure 7.8). In order to breathe, you have to twist your neck to one side. So here you are, sleeping or resting to reduce the effects of gravity and to give your body a well-deserved break, but your spine is twisted, creating more strain.

Sleeping on your stomach or in other strained sleeping postures are particularly significant because your body is supposed to relax. During sleep, the muscles and ligaments are not signaled to hold and protect the spine as much as when you are awake. Therefore, you are more vulnerable to excessive ligament and muscle strain from the contortions you put your body through during sleep. In addition, your body may not recognize that it is in a twisted position, and you may stay that way for longer periods of time than you would if you were awake. I mentioned in a previous chapter that muscle and ligament sprain and strain, and spinal misalignment can be caused by high forces on a joint over a short period of time or by low forces over a long period of time. It's the slow excessive or abnormal stretching through the course of your sleep, night after night, that can cause undesirable changes in your body and its balance and alignment, just as poor work postures strain you during the day. You can effectively reduce or eliminate these problems during sleep by using properly supportive bedding and adopting better sleeping postures.

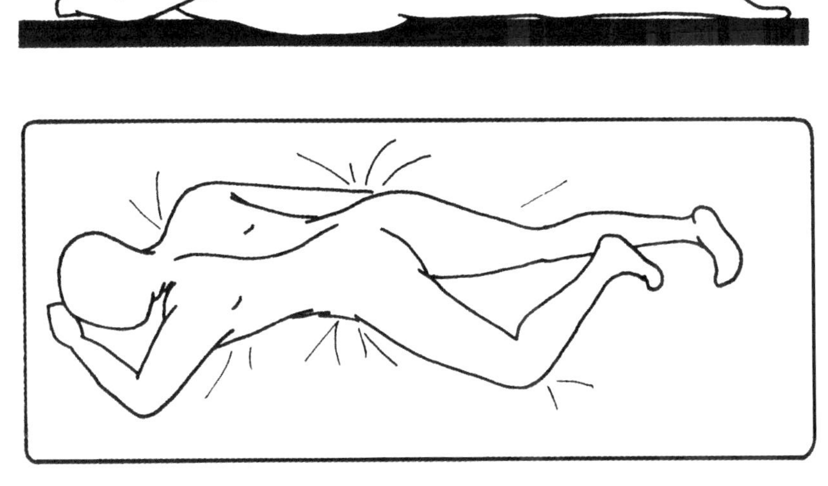

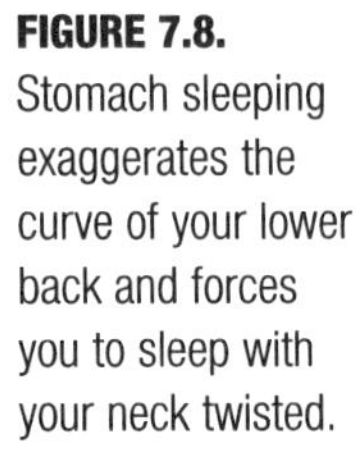

FIGURE 7.8. Stomach sleeping exaggerates the curve of your lower back and forces you to sleep with your neck twisted.

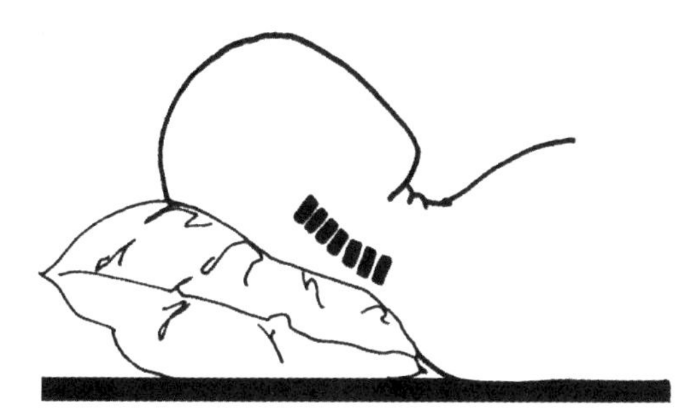

FIGURE 7.9. A thick pillow reduces the natural curve of your neck.

The two best sleeping postures are on your back or side. If you are already a back sleeper, you may not have much to worry about. Be sure, however, that you use your pillow properly. Remember that your neck should have a forward curve. If your pillow is thick, your head may rest on the pillow in a way that your neck is slightly flexed (see Figure 7.9). This position straightens or reverses the curve of your neck and pulls on the muscles and ligaments in back of your neck and upper back. If you combine this with the fact that your head may be frequently or continuously tilted forward during your workday and with the tensing effect of stress on these muscles, it's easy to understand why you may have muscle and ligament strain, spinal misalignment, or nerve irritation that cause neck and back pain and headaches. These problems also contribute to fatigue.

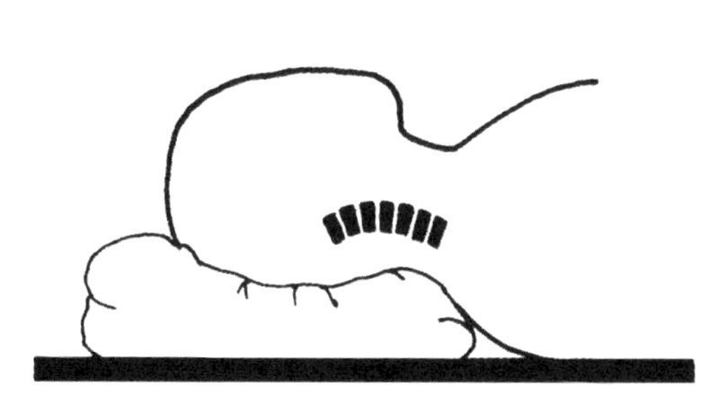

FIGURE 7.10. Specially designed pillows will support your neck in its proper position while sleeping on your back.

It is usually best to sleep on a thin pillow and curl it slightly under your neck so it supports your forward curve. Specially designed pillows that are contoured to properly support your neck and head are available (see Figure 7.10), and they are well worth the modest investment. It is very important to support your spine's natural curves during sleep. Seek professional guidance when selecting one of these special pillows.

Another major consideration for back sleepers is that it is not good to sleep for long periods of time with your arms above your head. This can put strain on your shoulders and upper arms as well as crowd the neck vertebrae and the muscles, ligaments, blood vessels, and nerves between your neck and shoulders, and can cause numbness and tingling in your arms and hands.

Many of us are side sleepers, and that's good too, but there are a few tricks

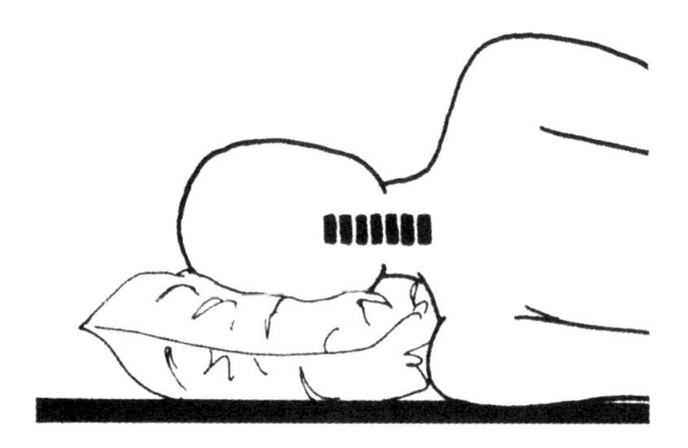

FIGURE 7.11. Your pillow should fill the space between your neck and the bed to keep your neck horizontal.

to proper side sleeping. Again, the pillow plays an important role. Your pillow should fill the space between your neck and the bed surface so that your neck is level with the bed (see Figure 7.11). If the pillow is too thin, your head and neck will bend toward the bed, and there will be crowding and jamming of the vertebrae on the side of your neck that is closest to the bed (see Figure 7.12). The shoulder on that same side may also be jammed. Meanwhile, the other side of your neck is stretched. If you sleep like this night after night, imbalance and misalignment, strain, and nerve irritation can occur, which contribute to or magnify the strains you encounter in your work and daily life. If your pillow is too thick while side sleeping, the side of your neck closest to the bed is stretched and the other side may be jammed (see Figure 7.13). A specially designed pillow can come to the rescue here as well, because it will support your neck so it is level with the bed's surface. Avoid sleeping with your arm under your neck and head. This can cause a problem similar to sleeping on your back with your arms overhead. Try to tuck your shoulder slightly forward with your forearm across your stomach or lying on the bed.

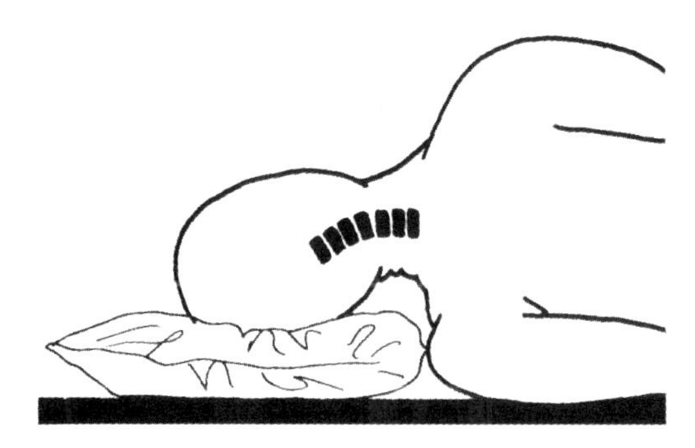

FIGURE 7.12. This pillow is too thin.

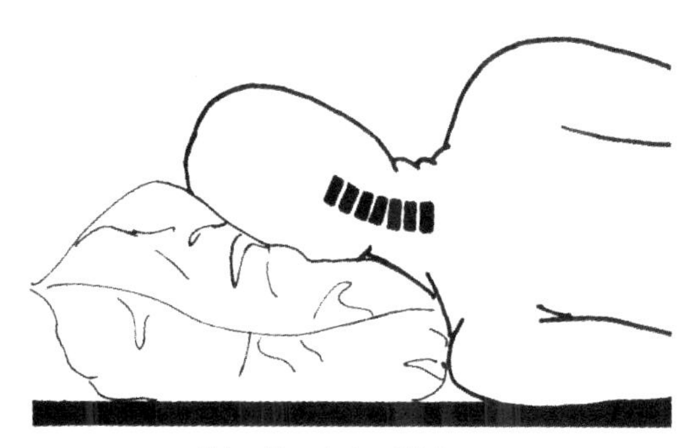

FIGURE 7.13. This pillow is too thick.

When you sleep on your side, your legs should be on top of each other with your knees bent. It's very easy to throw the top leg over toward the bed, but this makes your hips twist and rotates your pelvis and lower spine (see Figure 7.14). This strain, night after night, can cause the same type of strain for your lower back that a twisted or poorly supported neck can cause in your upper back. Try to keep your knees on top of each other (see Figure 7.15) or the upper knee slightly behind (see Figure 7.16). In many cases, it is acceptable to place a thin pillow between your knees, especially if you have bony knees and it's uncomfortable to keep them together.

Now you have the basics for good sleeping habits and postures. You have the ammunition to combat some of the problems that you may encounter with sleep and rest. All you have to do now is form the right habits. If you have problems changing some of your undesirable habits, be sure to study and apply the rules outlined for you in Chapter 8.

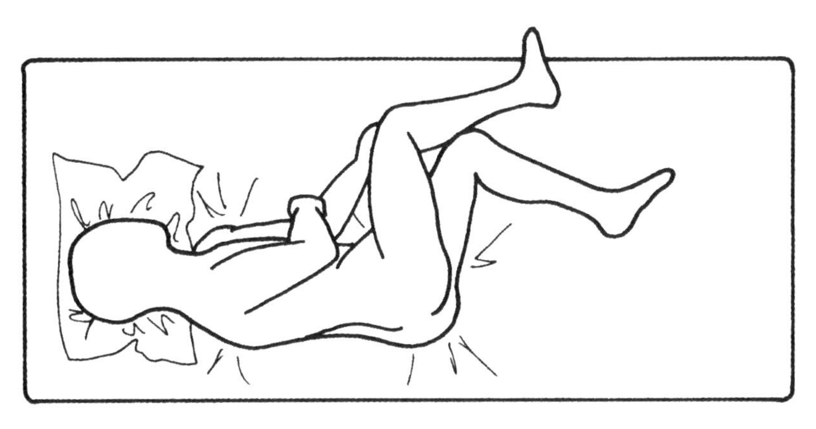

FIGURE 7.14. Sleeping with your top leg in front of your lower leg rotates your pelvis and twists your spine.

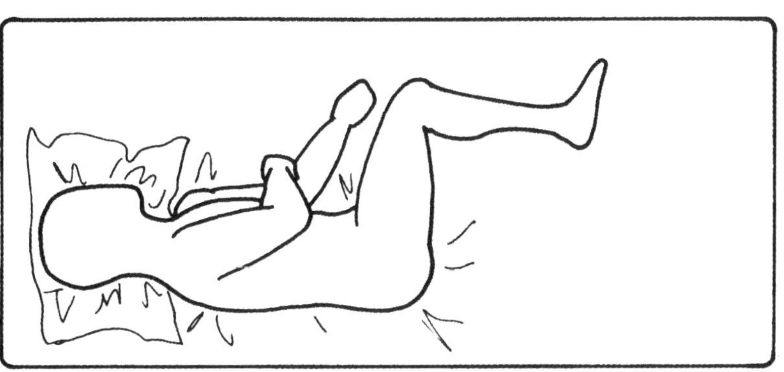

FIGURE 7.15. Place your knees directly on top of each other when sleeping on your side.

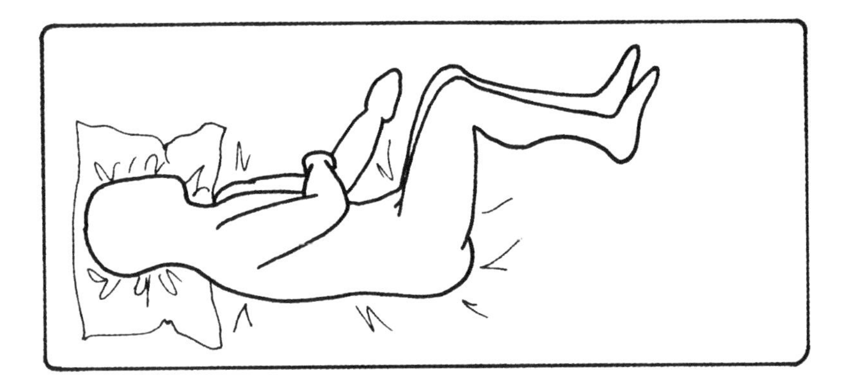

FIGURE 7.16. You may place the top knee slightly behind the other.

Caution

If you have had a neck or back condition or injury, you may be advised to sleep on your back with pillows under your knees and with your head, neck, and upper back supported with several pillows. You may even be advised to sleep partially on your stomach with several pillows to support you. These are special circumstances and the advice should be followed; however, after your injury has healed, these positions should not become your regular sleeping postures. Consult your doctor to determine if and when you can change to a different position.

Carefully follow the manufacturer's instructions and directions for sleeping on a specially designed cervical pillow. If you have trouble getting used to that type of pillow, seek professional advice. Inability to sleep with your body properly supported and positioned may be a warning sign that you have imbalance, misalignment, or abnormal movement in the joints of your spine, which may need to be corrected. Don't allow any questions to go unanswered.

People with heart or lung diseases, high blood pressure, and other conditions may not be able to sleep without special support. It is not the intent of this book to explain these particular circumstances. Therefore, if you have an unusual circumstance, it would be best to follow the appropriate recommendations of your personal healthcare professional.

8

Replacing Undesirable Habits

We are creatures of habit, and, over time, we tend to become creatures of our habits. If we form the habits of slumping (see Figure 8.1) or assuming awkward postures (see Figure 8.2), exercising very little, and allowing the effects of stress to accumulate in our bodies, without forming the habits required to counteract these changes, our bodies will become imbalanced, inflexible, tight, irritated, and fatigued. We will be more likely to suffer degeneration and ill health and miss the enjoyment we should experience in our lives both at work and at home.

Habits are usually learned responses that are acquired over time. They begin in the conscious mind and become programmed into the subconscious mind. After a habit has been learned by the subconscious, it becomes automatic or second nature because you don't have to consciously think about doing the habit. The routines we go through, day after day, are filled with minor and major habit patterns. To a large extent, we program the habits of our days. If you stop and think for a moment, it's amazing how much of our daily lives are built around our habits. If many of your habits are undesirable or bad for you, their effects will appear over a period of time. You may have unintentionally programmed the wrong responses into your subconscious mind. This causes

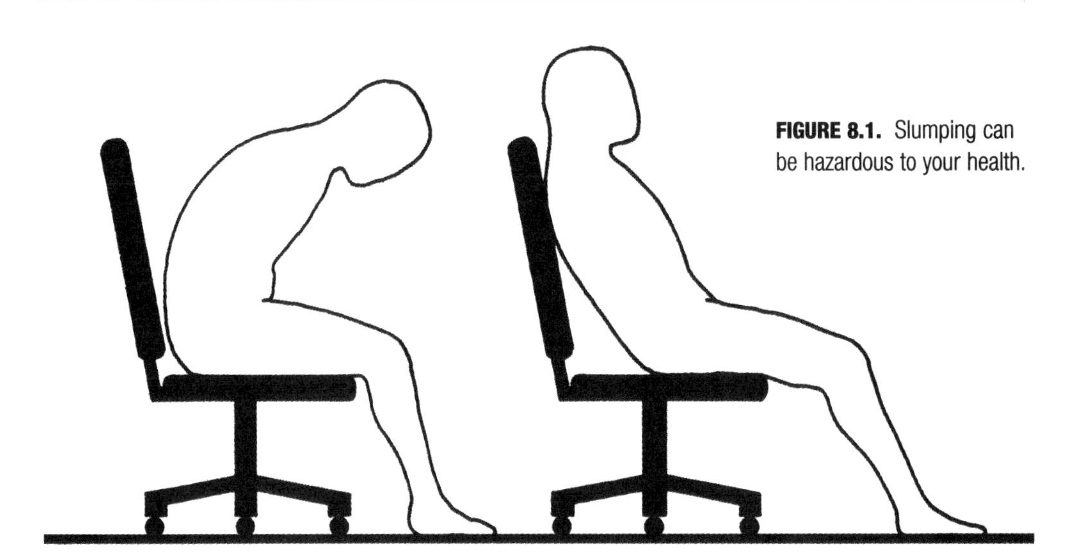

FIGURE 8.1. Slumping can be hazardous to your health.

you to respond the way you have conditioned yourself to feel and act, no matter how negative, false, distorted, or destructive it might be. Consequently, you must go through a period of unlearning or deprogramming in order to replace bad habits with a good habits.

By reading this book, you have a better understanding of how your body works, the way in which the unique circumstances of office work can adversely affect you, and many possible solutions to particular problems. You have learned how your workstation and chair should fit you, and how you need to properly fit your body to your workstation and chair. You know how factors in the work environment such as lighting, temperature, drafts, and noise can affect you, your job performance, and enjoyment, as well as ways to deal with them. You have learned how to properly sit for your particular task and how to ease or counteract the stress and strains you encounter (see Figure 8.3). You know that you need to "shift gears" during the day to escape the cumulative

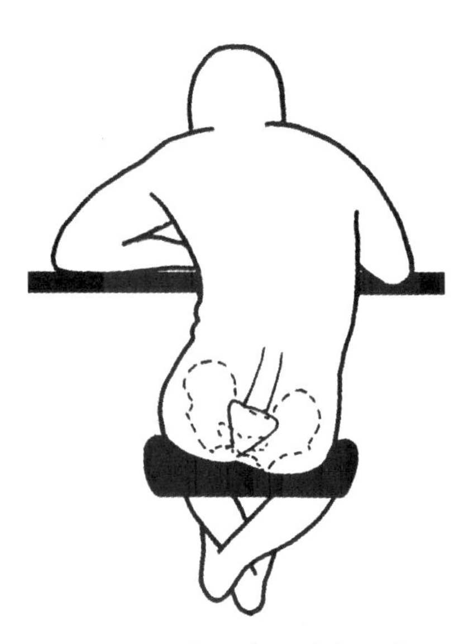

FIGURE 8.2. Assuming unbalanced postures creates strain on your body.

effects of stress on your body, shifting down through relaxation techniques (see Figure 8.4), and gearing up through enjoyable physical exercise (see Figure 8.5) to vent the pent-up energies within your body created by stress and the sedentary nature of your work. You've come to understand that your body must be kept flexible, well-balanced, and aligned or it may lose some of its capabilities and you will suffer problems and pain. You have read about many of the common symptoms sedentary workers experience, some of their causes, and how to improve or correct them. You even know how to sleep better.

It seems like so much to remember, but it's all extremely important to you and your well-being, as well as to your job performance and satisfaction. You should have this book nearby to refer to and always seek professional guidance if you have persistent problems or questions.

Many of the bad habits you have unintentionally formed should be now apparent to you, and it is to your benefit to take action to replace them with good habits. This takes work, but if you use the following advice, you can do it. Don't be discouraged if you have many habits to change. Most of us do! The most important thing is to simply get started. It will take time and effort, but the rewards will be well worth it.

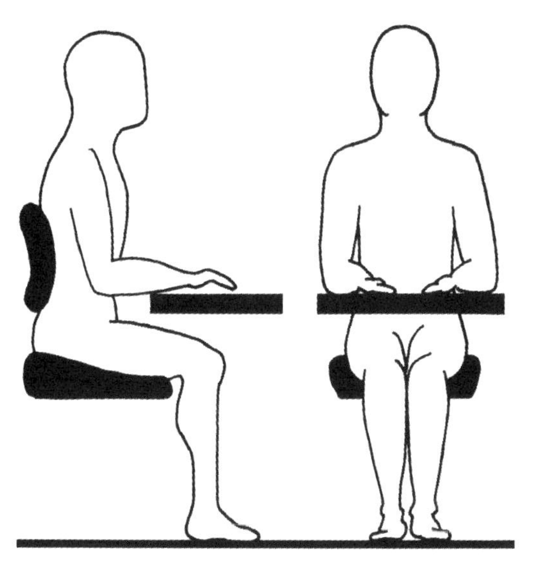

FIGURE 8.3. Practice good postural habits at work and at home.

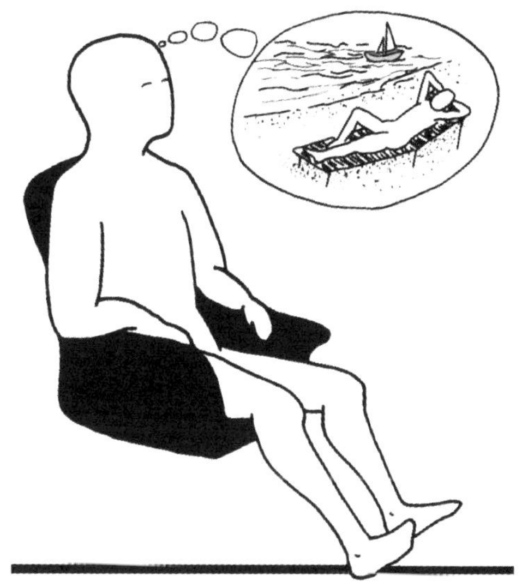

FIGURE 8.4. Shift to a lower gear to relax from the effects of stress.

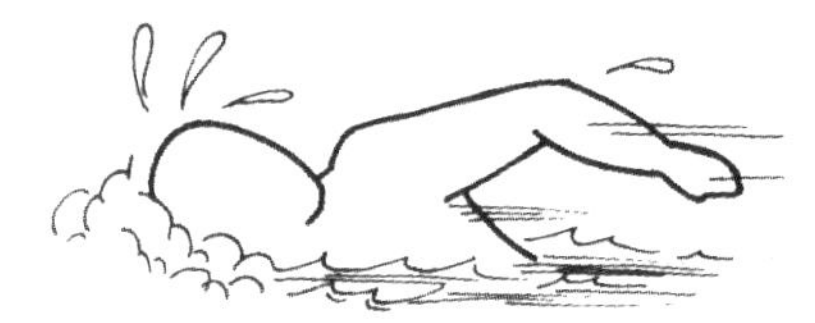

FIGURE 8.5. Shift to a higher gear to physically vent stress.

No amount of willpower is of any use unless we really want to give up old habits. Most of the time we want to give up the painful effects of our habits, but are not willing to do what it takes to give up the habits themselves. If you feel you are being forced to replace a bad habit with a good one, you will start feeling deprived or that you are sacrificing too much. This creates negative feelings such as guilt, frustration, and anxiety, as well as stress, which make it impossible to change for more than a short time. It's a matter of attitude. You have to be "sold" on the idea and be motivated by the benefits you will receive. Do not condemn yourself for having bad habits or condemn the habits themselves. Accept the fact that you have a bad habit that you want to replace with a good habit. Becoming angry with yourself can also cause the negative feelings that produce resistance to change.

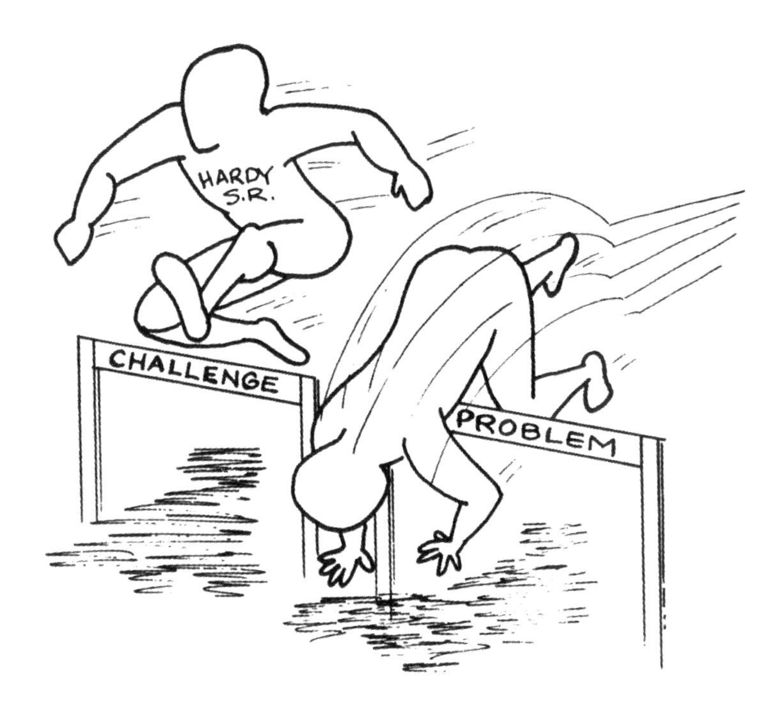

FIGURE 8.6. Changing undesirable habits is a challenge, not a problem.

Make a list of the habits you want to change. This will allow you to keep track of them and enable you to check your progress. It is a personal list and you do not have to show it to anyone unless you want to. Next, jot down how you are going to change those habits or which desirable habits you are going to replace them with. Write down the easiest and most logical way to accomplish this. Visualize yourself as already having succeeded in changing your habits. See yourself enjoying the benefits of your new positive habits. Pat yourself on the back for taking the necessary actions to accomplish your goals. Observe your actions and note every time you fail to do what you promised yourself. Remember, do not condemn or scold yourself. Simply make an objective observation and allow yourself to make the necessary correction. Keep a record for at least twenty-one days. You are actually using conscious thought and action to retrain your subconscious mind so the new habits will become automatic or second nature. You can train your conscious and subconscious thoughts, just as you can physically train or exercise your body to get in shape. It may be difficult at first, but it gets easier if you stick with your program.

You can promise yourself anything, but keep in mind that the important thing is to make the commitment to replace the bad habits with good habits. Start now! Don't put it off. Once you are successful in changing a habit, you not only gain the benefits of the more desirable habit, but you will also begin to gain in self-confidence by knowing that you are improving yourself. You may even build up some of that enthusiasm for working and enjoying life that may have dwindled over the years.

Conclusion

The Choice Is Yours!

Knowledge, action, and consistency are the keys that unlock the doors for a brighter, healthier future for you. Yes, you can learn not only to survive but also to thrive in your chosen occupation. You have been provided with much of the knowledge you need to understand your body, your workstation, as well as methods for taking action to improve yourself and your surroundings. It is up to you to use this knowledge and act accordingly to enhance the quality of your life and your work. It is critically important that you be consistent in your efforts. Without consistent action, you will fall back into the ruts you were in before.

The road to health and happiness is a journey, not a destination. Consistent positive action will make your journey through life more pleasant and fulfilling. It's your choice. Do you want to merely exist and survive, or thrive and enjoy?

Appendix A

PERSONAL LIFESTYLE INVENTORY

The quality of your life is in your hands! In order to determine what measures you should take to improve your level of positive wellness, you must have an idea of the status of your current lifestyle. Circle the appropriate answers to the following questions in the brief *Personal Lifestyle Inventory.* Score your answers according to the directions on page 122 to gain an understanding of where you stand. The *Personal Lifestyle Inventory* was organized and developed by Thomas M. Wolff, APR, an editor for the Foundation For Chiropractic Education and Research.

PERSONAL LIFESTYLE INVENTORY

Circle answer a, b, or c for each question. Give yourself five points for each "a" answer, three points for each "b" answer, and one point for each "c" answer. Record the section total where indicated.

GENERAL

1. How do you rate your own health and vitality compared with that of others your age and sex?

a) extremely healthy, very energetic

b) about average health and energy

c) in poor health, tired a lot

2. Do you use tobacco?

a) no

b) smoke fewer than 10 cigarettes or 5 cigars a day

c) smoke more than that 10 cigarettes or 5 cigars a day

3. Do you drink alcohol?

a) 0–7 drinks a week

b) 8–15 drinks a week

c) more than 15 drinks a week
(A "drink" is 1.25 ounces of hard liquor, 12 ounces of beer, or 4 ounces of wine.)

4. Do you wear a seatbelt when driving or riding in a car?

a) always **b)** sometimes **c)** never

5. Do you seek professional attention from your doctor of chiropractic or other physician when you have symptoms or conditions that need checking?

a) always **b)** sometimes **c)** never

General subtotal: ________

STRESS

6. Do tension and worries interfere with your daily activities or relationships or contribute to headaches or pain in the neck, shoulders, or back?

a) seldom

b) occasionally

c) frequently

7. Do you use tranquilizer drugs or alcohol in attempts to relieve tension?

a) never **b)** sometimes **c)** frequently

8. Do you take time each day to quiet your mind and relax your body?

a) yes **b)** sometimes **c)** never

9. How many hours of restful sleep do you get each night?

a) 6–8 hours b) more than 9

c) fewer than 5

10. Do you cope with stress by such methods as setting realistic goals, building close relationships, recreation, humor, and exercise?

a) yes, generally b) some of these

c) no

Stress subtotal: ________

NUTRITION

11. Are you overweight or underweight?

a) no b) by 5–19 pounds

c) by 20 or more pounds

12. Does your daily diet include something from each of the four basic food groups: (1) meats, fish, poultry, eggs, dried legumes, nuts; (2) milk and milk products; (3) whole-grain bread and cereals; (4) fruits and vegetables?

a) each day

b) three times weekly

c) seldom

13. Do you limit your fat and salt intake?

a) vegetables, fruits, lean meat only, no extra salt

b) meat, eggs, cheese 12–24 times weekly, little salt

c) meat, cheese, eggs, whole milk, snacks more than 24 times weekly, lots of salt

14. Do you limit sugar and have enough fiber intake?

a) whole-grain cereals, fruits and vegetables, almost no sugar

b) mixed whole grain and white breads, fruits and vegetables, little sugar

c) heavy on desserts, sugar, white breads, low on fruits and vegetables

15. Do you eat a breakfast that contains a third of your daily need for calories, proteins, and vitamins?

a) a great deal

b) three times a week

c) seldom or never

Nutrition subtotal: ________

EXERCISE

16. How much physical effort do you expend on your job and other physical activities (such as housework and yard work)?

a) a great deal

b) moderate amount

c) very little

17. Do you participate in vigorous physical exercise?

a) at least a half hour, three times a week

b) once a week

c) occasionally or never
("Vigorous exercise" will cause you to perspire and your pulse will be above 120.)

18. What is the average number of miles you walk briskly, jog, or run per day?

a) more than a mile

b) less than a mile

c) virtually none

19. Do you climb up and down stairs and walk instead of drive, when feasible?

a) usually

b) occasionally

c) never

20. Do you stretch and bend a few minutes each day to keep your body flexible?

a) usually

b) occasionally

c) never

Exercise subtotal: ________

Grand total: ________

SCORING AND INTERPRETATION

Add up the subtotals for the four sections to get your grand total. For interpretation of your score, read below.

If you have a total score of 90–100, you rate "excellent." You have a strong awareness of sensible lifestyle habits in all areas and you practice them.

If you have a total score of 75–89, your ranking is "good." You are above average, and with minimum improvements, you could be excellent.

If you have a total score of 61–74, your ranking is "not so good." You have a number of lifestyle habits that are potential health problems.

If you have a total score below 60, you are in a risk area. With effort, you can modify your habits and overcome potential health hazards.

Appendix B

NUTRITIONAL CONSIDERATIONS

There are many theories and philosophies concerning nutrition. This section is provided to give you an overview of the basic concepts involved in a balanced diet. Certain health conditions may require special nutritional considerations so do not hesitate to seek professional assistance.

Sedentary workers differ from their heavy labor counterparts not only in their tasks, but also in their nutritional requirements. Heavy labor occupations involving much physical exertion may require workers to consume 3,000 to 5,000 calories per day. People who earn their livings while sitting use less physical energy so their calorie expenditure may be only 2,000 to 3,000 calories per day. Consequently, sedentary workers should be more concerned about the quality of their food intake than the quantity. It is advisable to cut down on energy-rich and highly refined or processed foods in favor of more natural foods such as vegetables, fruits, whole-grain breads, natural dairy products, and lean meats.

With this in mind, let's review some basic concepts about nutrition. In 1985, the U.S. Department of Agriculture and the U.S. Department of Health and Human Services issued the following revised dietary guidelines:

1. Eat a variety of foods.

2. Maintain a desirable weight.
3. Avoid too much fat, saturated fat, and cholesterol.
4. Eat foods with adequate starch and fiber.
5. Avoid too much sugar.
6. Avoid too much sodium (salt).
7. If you drink alcoholic beverages, do so in moderation.

The foods and liquids that you eat, digest, and assimilate build and maintain all of the cells of your body and provide the energy you need to live and work. If you do not give your body the proper nutrients and fuel for energy, you cannot have and maintain good health. You should therefore strive for a balanced diet that includes the four basic food groups (fruits and vegetables; breads, grains, and cereals; protein; and dairy products) plus one other essential element, water.

Fruits and vegetables provide healthy complex carbohydrates for energy, plus fiber and minerals, as well as A, B, and C vitamins. At least four servings a day from this group is recommended.

Whole-grain or enriched bread, cooked or dry cereal, pasta, rice, oats, and corn also provide healthy complex carbohydrates plus B vitamins, protein, iron, and fiber. Four servings a day from this group is also recommended.

Lean meats, poultry, fish, eggs, dry beans, nuts, seeds, peanut butter, and soy products provide protein, essential amino acids, fat, iron, fiber, and A, B, and E vitamins. Two servings a day is recommended.

Dairy products provide calcium and amino acids, and are often enriched to provide vitamin D. Adult men require two servings a day but adult women and children should have four servings a day. Low-fat dairy products are usually preferable.

An essential element that is often neglected is water. Water not only refreshes the fluids of our bodies, but it is also essential in many of the chemical reactions that are required for life. Under normal circumstances, our bodies need one ounce of water for each two pounds of body weight every day. For instance, if you weigh 128 pounds, you should drink one gallon (64 ounces) of water each day. Coffee, tea, and other beverages are not an adequate substitute for fresh water. Do not take this concept to an extreme and drink a large quantity of other fluids such as coffee, tea, colas, or other beverages in addition to the amount of water you should be drinking. Certain health conditions such as high blood pressure and kidney, heart, or lung problems may require limited fluid intake. Consult a qualified health professional, if needed, before you increase your water consumption.

The best source of nutrition comes from natural, unprocessed foods, but we live in an era in which highly processed and preserved foods are so easy to obtain that they readily become a major source of our food intake. For this reason, nutritional supplements may help fulfill your needs. If you go into a health food store and look around, you will see shelves full of various vitamins, minerals, and other items that report to be just what you need. This can be confusing, and you may not know what would be best for you. Consult a healthcare professional who is knowledgeable in nutrition to help you understand what you need.

Appendix C

BACKLESS SEATING AND OTHER SEATING INNOVATIONS

One of the most frequent questions asked when I am speaking to groups of office workers about chairs concerns the Balans or kneeling chair. As you can see from the illustration on this page, the Balans chair represents an intriguing new concept in chair design. One of the major theories is that when the thighs angle downward to this degree, the curve of the lower back more easily assumes its natural position. I have sat in several of these chairs and personally find them to be very comfortable. I have not, however, used this chair for extended periods of time. I have not discovered any research that addresses the effects of this type of chair on the long-term, high-frequency user.

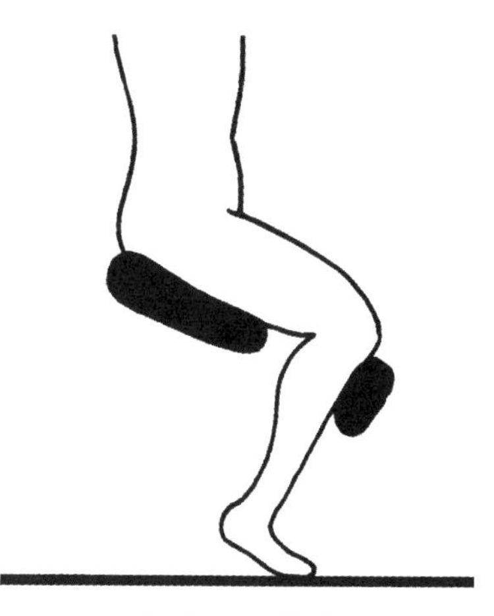

The Balans Chair

Areas of possible concern are the effects on the circulation in the legs and feet; the effects of prolonged knee pressure applied from the kneeling pads; the effects on the ankles and feet in the positions they are maintained; and the adjustability of the chair to fit a wide range of workstations and tasks. (For example, can you safely and comfortably bend, twist, and reach in the various positions your tasks require while you are using this type of chair?) One other area of concern is the chair's capacity to allow the user to assume the three common sitting postures discussed in Chapter 2 (work-intensive, conversational, and relaxation). The use of this type of chair may require a higher work surface in order to keep from slumping forward. This would present a problem if your workstation was not adjustable. If a person utilizing this type of chair begins to experience leg, knee, ankle, foot, or other symptoms from its use, they should obtain a different chair and consult a qualified healthcare professional.

Clearly, this type of seating has its advantages in helping many people sit more comfortably and correctly. I have seen patients with significant back problems become more comfortable and productive from its use. Whether it fits you and your tasks requires careful consideration and evaluation. Its future use and popularity will be interesting to watch.

Dr. Brock Walker's ENGINEERED SEATING SOLUTIONS are implemented in several user-friendly forms for all parts of our lives. Dr. Walker is an expert in enhancing human performance and successfully treating musculoskeletal problems. After a series of personal injuries, he turned to designing seating, and his research and engineering solutions have already been used in the aerospace and motorsports industries. One of his most successful solutions was for Buddy Lazier after a serious accident in 1996 had left the race-car driver with multiple spinal fractures and unable to stand, sit, or lay down without experiencing excruciating pain. The safe, supportive seat that Dr. Walker designed for Buddy's race car allowed him to compete in, and WIN, the grueling Indianapolis 500. If Dr. Walker can ameliorate such a dire condition, imagine what he can do for the rest of us.

Appendix D

CORPORATE AND INDIVIDUAL SOLUTIONS

As you read this book, you will become more aware of yourself and your surroundings. You will also undoubtedly discover aspects of your environment, such as automobile seats, beds, pillows, and chairs, to name a few, that do not fit you properly, so you may want to contact Peak Health & Safety for individual questions or help.

Like individuals, companies frequently have challenges with health and safety issues affecting their employees. Also, just as individuals who do not pay attention to their habits will not usually enjoy a peak-performance life, companies that do not pay attention to employee health and safety circumstances will not enjoy peak corporate performance and profitability. Corporate needs are best assessed and dealt with using a variety of products and services, including the ones we offer.

Whether you have individual or corporate needs, you can contact us at our website, www.peakhealthandsafety.com. You can also call our message and order center at 1-800-552-6347 (U.S. only) to ask questions or request information. Here are a few of the services and products that can help both individuals and companies.

SERVICES

All services described below can be accessed through our website.

- ❑ We have developed a remarkable CLOSED-LOOP COMPUTER-BASED TRAINING PROGRAM to accelerate the learning process outlined in this book, and it is designed to automatically adjust to your own pace.

- ❑ BIONOMICS is a new term developed through Future Industrial Technologies by its president, Dennis Downing. It is a field related to ergonomics that combines the teaching of biomechanics, posture, and non-strenuous stretching. The goal of Bionomics is to teach, through proper body management, how to prevent the occurrence of physical stress in the first place or, if there is already physical stress present, how to relieve the body of any accumulation of it. This training, known as *BACKSAFE™* and *SITTINGSAFE™*, is performed in small group settings conducted by one of more than 1,100 trained facilitators throughout North America. If companies comply with the recommendations made during the initial assessment and the subsequent phases of the program, they can usually reduce the incidence and/or cost of work injuries by 40 to 70 percent. Participants learn how to be responsible for their own physical well-being, both on and off the job. *BACKSAFE* and *SITTINGSAFE* training both complement the information in this book, and both are excellent ways to effectively transform your habits with professional guidance.

- ❑ We offer CORPORATE HEALTH AND SAFETY MANAGEMENT, and can customize solutions for you based on our analysis of the needs and risks involved We work with several organizations, including the ACA Council on Occupational Health, and the related IACOHC, that can offer additional solutions.

- ❑ Our MOTIVATIONAL WORKSHOPS AND SEMINARS, based on our unique and prevention-oriented concepts, are specifically designed to achieve practical results.

- ❑ For personal and corporate applications, we can EVALUATE AN INDIVIDUAL'S PHYSICAL CAPACITY AND PERFORMANCE using high-tech methods.

- The subject is beyond the scope of this book, but we have now made information available on PROPER NUTRITION, SUPPLEMENTATION, AND WATER, which are essential components for a peak performance body and mind.

PRODUCTS

All products and guidelines below can be accessed through our website.

- The *BACK FLEX*™ HEALTHY BACK SYSTEM is an innovative method for relieving back strain while improving posture. Regular use can relieve back pain, slumping, and stress, and can increase the users' awareness of how to adjust their own chairs, desks, seats, etc. to fit better for good posture.

- We can provide CD-ROM-BASED INTERACTIVE VIDEO PROGRAMS ON HEALTH AND SAFETY. The routines are specifically designed for improved balance, flexibility, posture, strength, and stress management. These kits also include printed material, Swiss exercise balls or exercise tubing, and are very user-friendly and portable.

- INNOVATIVE CUSHIONS, PILLOWS, SUPPORTS, AND WEDGES are available here or through links we can provide to other sources. Made from a variety of materials, all are designed to help match your unique form and needs to your environment and the tasks you perform.

- We have GUIDELINES FOR PURCHASING everything from clothing to vehicles, which are based on how well the item would fit in terms of its function, fashion, and value.

References

Anderson, B., *Stretching*. Shelter Publications, Inc., Bolinas, CA, 1980.

Andersson, B.J.G., "The Sitting Posture, an Electromyographic and Discometric Study." *Orthopedic Clinics of North America*, Vol. 6, No. 1, 1975, pp. 105–120.

Arndt, R., "Ergonomic Considerations in Office Design." National Office Products Association, Alexandria, VA, 1976.

AT&T-Bell Laboratories, *Video Display Terminals: Preliminary Guidelines for Selection, Installation and Use*. Bell Telephone Laboratories, Inc., 1983,

Bendix, T., "Seat Inclination and Trunk Posture." Laboratory for Back Research, Department of Rheumatology, Rigshospitalet, University of Copenhagen, Denmark, 1985.

Cetron, M., and O'Toole, T., *Encounters with the Future, A Forecast of Life into the Twenty-first Century*. McGraw-Hill, New York, 1982.

Charlesworth, E.A., and Nathan, R. G., *Stress Management: A Comprehensive Guide to Wellness*. Ballantine Books, New York, 1984.

Christensen, K., *Clinical Chiropractic Biomechanics*. Foot Levelers, Inc., Dubuque, IA, 1984.

Christensen, K., *Clinical Chiropractic Orthopedics*. Foot Levelers, Inc., Des Moines, IA, 1984.

Cousins, N., *Anatomy of an Illness.* W. W. Norton and Company, New York, 1979.

Fahrni, H., *Backache Assessment and Treatment.* Musqueam Publishers, Vancouver, B.C., Canada, 1975.

Flesia, J., and Reikeman, R., *A Psycho-Epistemological Basis for the New Renaissance Intellectual.* Renaissance International, Colorado Springs, CO, 1981.

Foundation for Chiropractic Education and Research, "How Chiropractic Fits Your Fitness." Staying Well, Des Moines, IA, May–June, 1985. Foundation for Chiropractic Education and Research, "How to Relax and Enjoy It." *Staying Well,* Des Moines, IA, November December, 1985.

Foundation for Chiropractic Education and Research, "How to Save Your Neck." *Staying Well,* Des Moines, IA, July–August, 1985.

Foundation for Chiropractic Education and Research, "How to Survive and Thrive with Stress." *Staying Well,* Des Moines, IA, January–February, 1985.

Foundation for Chiropractic Education and Research, "It's the Way You Handle Stress." *Staying Well,* Des Moines, IA, July August, 1985.

Foundation for Chiropractic Education and Research, "Limber Up By Stretching." *Staying Well,* Des Moines, IA, May–June, 1986.

Foundation for Chiropractic Education and Research, "Move It: A Major Key to Your Wellness." *Staying Well,* March–April, 1985.

Foundation for Chiropractic Education and Research, "Sleep: It's the Quality, Not the Quantity." *Staying Well,* Des Moines, IA, November–December, 1983.

Foundation for Chiropractic Education and Research, "Tailoring Your Exercise Plans to Mt." *Staying Well,* Des Moines, IA, September–October, 1985.

Foundation for Chiropractic Education and Research, "The Whys and Hows of Fitness." *Staying Well,* Des Moines, IA, March–April, 1986.

Foundation for Chiropractic Education and Research, "What You Can Eat to Help You Stay Well." *Staying Well,* Des Moines, IA, January–February, 1986.

Goss, C., *Gray's Anatomy.* Lea and Febiger, Philadelphia, 1973.

Grandjean, E., *Ergonomics of the Home.* Taylor and Francis Ltd, London, 1973.

Grandjean, E., *Fitting the Task to the Man: An Ergonomic Approach.* Taylor and Francis Inc., Philadelphia, 1980.

Guyton, A.C., *Textbook of Medical Physiology.* W. B. Saunders Company, Philadelphia, 1981.

Herman Miller, Inc., "Ergon Chairs: Healthful, Supportive Seating for a Wide Range of Work Activities." Zeeland, Michigan, 1982.

Hittleman, R., *Introduction to Yoga: Beginning and Intermediate Exercises for Peace and Physical Fulfillment.* Bantam Books, Inc., New York, NY, 1977.

Hoppenfield, S., *Physical Examination of the Spine and Extremities.* Appleton-Century-Crofts, New York, 1976.

Hughes, PC., and McNelis, J.F, "Lighting, Productivity, and the Work Environment." *Lighting Design and Application,* December, 1978, pp. 32–39.

International Academy of Chiropractic Industrial Consultants, Lectures and notes from the "Chiropractic Industrial Consultant Certificate Program." sponsored by Northwestern College of Chiropractic, Bloomington, MN, and The Iowa Chiropractic Society, Des Moines, IA, September 1984–June 1985.

International Business Machines Corporation, *Human Factors of Workstations with Visual Displays.* IBM, 1984.

Jan, H.H., *The 1986 Success Journal.* Jan Associates, Piedmont, CA, 1981.

Knight, E.L., *Flexibility: The Concept of Stretching and Exercise.* Kendall-Hunt, Dubuque, IA, 1984.

Kobasa, S.O., and Maddi, S.A., *The Hardy Executive: Health Under Stress.* Dow Jones-Irwin, 1984.

Krueger, Inc. (with Emilio Ambasz) "Seating Systems, Fatigue and Productivity." Green Bay, WI, 1984.

Krueger, Inc. (with Emilio Ambasz) "The Principles of Office Chair Selection." Green Bay, WI, 1984.

Krueger, Inc. (with Emilio Ambasz), "Vertebra vs. the Backache Syndrome." Green Bay, WI, 1984.

Leach, R.A., and Phillips, R.B., *The Chiropractic Theories: A Synopsis of Scientific Research.* Williams & Wilkins, Baltimore, 1985.

Lueder, R.K., *The Ergonomics Payoff. A Guide to Designing the Electronic Office.* Holt, Rinehart and Winston, Toronto, 1986.

Maltz, M., *Psycho-Cybernetics.* Simon and Schuster, 1969.

Mayo, E., *The Human Problems of an Industrial Civilization.* The Macmillan Company, New York, 1938.

McNelis, J.F, "Human Performance—A Pilot Study." *Journal of the IES,* April, 1973, pp. 190–196.

Nachmenson, A., "Intravital Dynamic Pressure Measurements in Lumbar Discs." *Scandinavian Journal of Rehabilitation Medicine,* R Suppl. 1, 1970.

Naisbitt, J., *Megatrends: Ten New Directions Transforming Our Lives.* Warner Books, Inc., New York, NY, 1984.

Naisbitt, J., and Aburdene, P., *Reinventing The Corporation: Transforming Your Job and Your Company for the New Information Society.* Warner Books, Inc., New York, NY, 1985.

Pearce, R.B., "Working with VDT's: The Human Interface." Krames Communications, Daly City, CA 1984.

Ross, K.C., "A Guide to Managing Stress." Krames Communications, Daly City, CA, 1985.

Sauter, S.L., *Improving VDT Work: Causes and Control of Health Concerns in VDT Use."* The University of Wisconsin Board of Regents, Reprinted by permission and distributed by The Report Store, Lawrence, KS.

Selye, H., *Stress Without Distress.* Lippincott, Philadelphia, 1974.

Semente, R.A., and Karle, E.J., "The Effects of Manipulative Therapy on Arthritis and Neuromusculoskeletal Pain Disorders." *ACA Journal of Chiropractic,* Vol. 18, September 1984, pp. 67–75.

Sportelli, L., *Introduction to Chiropractic: A Natural Method of Health Care.* Louis Sportelli, D.C., Palmerton, PA, 1983.

Therapeutic Products, "Sleep and Plastic Deformation on Connective Tissue in Relationship to Kinetic Joint Stability and Integrity of the Cervical Spine." *Research Bulletin,* No. 617, Dubuque, IA, 1985.

United States Department of Health and Human Services, *Health Issues—Video Display Terminals.* May, 1984.

Ward, C., and Landis, K., Landis Ward Management, Danville, CA, Lecture Notes on "Positive Habit Reconditioning Program." February, 1984.

Webster's Seventh New Collegiate Dictionary. C. & G. Merriam Company, Springfield, Mass., 1967.

Wolf, M.D., "The Office Report: A Quick Fix for Office Tension." *Bruce Jenner's Better Health and Living,* April, 1986, pp. 60–63.

Ziglar, Z., *See You at the Top.* Pelican Publishing Company, Gretna, LA, 1981.

Index

I

J

K

L

M

N

P

R